Wolfgang Rosenbauer

Better Vision
Naturally

Simple Daily Exercises to Improve Your Eyesight

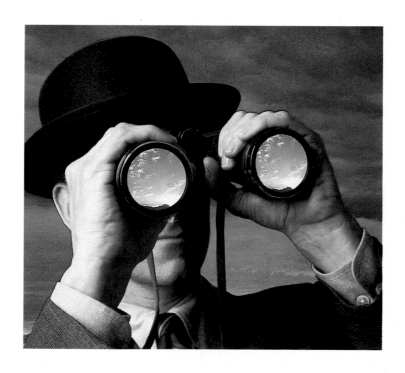

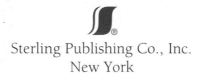

Sterling Publishing Co., Inc.
New York

Library of Congress Cataloging-in-Publication Data

Hatcher-Rosenbauer, Wolfgang.
  [Augenschule fur gesundes Sehen. English]
  Better vision naturally: simple daily exercises to improve you eyesight / Wolfgang Hatscher-Rosenbauer.
      p.   cm.
  Includes index.
  ISBN 0-8069-9981-0
  1. Visual training. 2. Orthoptics. I. Title.
RE960. H37713   1998
617.7—dc21   98–19655
                                   CIP

10 9 8 7 6 5 4 3 2 1

Published by Sterling Publishing
    Company, Inc.
    387 Park Avenue South, New York, N.Y. 10016
Corrected edition published and
    © 1996 in Germany by Südwest
    Verlag GmbH & Co. KG, Munich
    under the title *Augenschule für gesundes Sehen*
English translation © 1998 by Sterling
    Publishing Co., Inc.
Distributed in Canada by Sterling
    Publishing
    % Canadian Manda Group,
    One Atlantic Avenue, Suite 105
    Toronto, Ontario, Canada M6K 3E7
Distributed in Great Britain and Europe
    by Cassell PLC
    Wellington House,
    125 Strand, London WC2R 0BB,
    England
Distributed in Australia by Capricorn
    Link (Australia) Pty Ltd.
    P.O. Box 6651, Baulkham Hills,
    Business Centre, NSW 2153,
    Australia
Manufactured in the United States of America
Sterling ISBN 0-8069-9981-0

Contents

Healthy Tips for the Eyes 58

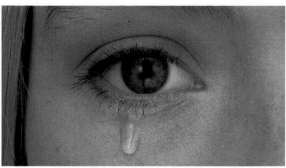

Emotions can influence vision.

Disadvantages of Visual Aids 66

Eye Training with Posters 70

Exercising Your Perception of Contrast 71

Short Exercises for Lively Vision 89

Index 96

Introduction

We rarely realize how important our eyesight is until we begin to lose vision or until we injure one of our eyes.

The goal of eye training is to try to improve the health of our eyes, to increase visual acuity, and to prevent mistakes or problems before they occur. The author developed this concept as part of a seminar dealing with preventive medicine. Since 1992, the agency that insures employees of the city of Frankfurt has accepted this as a method of treatment and prevention. In addition, large industrial companies have used it with great success.

Usually, course participants are people whose eyes face a great deal of stress, such as prolonged computer work, intense and concentrated reading, and work with monotonous and repetitive data. All of these can be stressful for the eyes. In addition, insufficient lighting, limited eye movement, and a lack of physical activity often intensify the stress. The lack of physical movement interferes with blood circulation in the visual center of the brain.

Results of Eye Training

➥ Short term: Reduces symptoms of visual stress, such as burning eyes, headaches, lack of concentration, and mental, as well as physical, exhaustion.

➥ Long term: Stabilizes and improves existing visual abilities. Some individuals can even reduce the strength of their prescription glasses because of their improved vision and visual accuity.

Good eyesight is a precious gift. We can do much to preserve and protect it.

Eye Training as Prevention

As early as the beginning of this century, ophthalmologists knew that glasses were not a cure-all for visual defects, poor eyesight, or defective vision. They recommended that people train their eyes to prevent eyestrain and bad habits. However, eye specialists find it difficult to include eye exercise instructions in their examinations. Furthermore, emotional and mental factors can contribute to visual problems. Since most eye doctors are not trained in mental health, the concept of exercising the eyes is still not part of their repertoire.

What Is Eye Training?

As we mentioned, doctors developed the idea of exercising the eyes with prevention in mind. In this book, we discuss the concept in four parts:

➡ The material from five lessons that deal with coordinating and strengthening vision (see pages 18 to 57).
➡ Helpful suggestions for better eye health, including simple and effective preventive measures from natural medicine and alternative visual aids for supporting sight (see pages 58 to 69).
➡ Eight exercise posters for training visual behavior, also helpful for developing proper visual habits (see pages 70 to 88).
➡ Twenty short exercises that are easy to learn and take only a few minutes (see pages 89 to 94).

Even if you only do the short exercises on a daily basis, they will enable you, at least temporarily, to relax your eyes and free new visual energies.

During the 1930s, Dr. William Bates, an American ophthalmologist, attempted to heal all visual defects without corrective lenses. While his ideas were very controversial, they were considered effective.

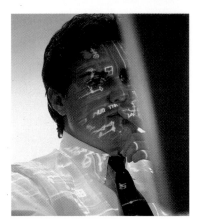

Working in front of a computer screen for hours at a time is extremely stressful for your eyes.

The fact that much of the visual process is not instinctive but learned was a revolutionary discovery.

Vision and Eye Training Today

Radical scientific advancement often takes place only in interdisciplinary areas. Ecology, biophysics, biochemistry, quantum physics, quantum electrodynamics, and other areas have developed an expanding, holistic picture of the material world, changing our view of it.

Today's new humanism, science and psychotherapy, the intercultural dialogue, the meeting of East and West and of North and South are also constantly changing the holistic image we have of ourselves. A program dedicated to the care of our eyes should not lag behind.

Understanding Vision

Our understanding of health is undergoing a change. Not so long ago, health meant the absence of illness, but today's holistic medicine defines health in terms of preventing illness, and prevention is each individual's responsibility. Today, health also refers to the quality of life, a process of growth on the emotional and mental level. Our understanding human vision is likewise undergoing an evolutionary process. Today, we believe that we can change and train vision. We've learned to "see" in a particular way, but that way is constantly changing, in the same way that, over time, human vision has adapted to the constantly changing demands of the environment. For instance, the amount and speed of visual information transmitted through the modern media is constantly expanding.

This development can have positive effects. For example, according to recent research, the ability of the human brain to deal with the increasing amount of "input" is actually expanding.

Eyeglasses or Contact Lenses Alone Won't Do

In spite of the obvious advances in ophthalmology and optometry, more and more people suffer from visual defects.

Studies conducted during the last fourteen years show that fifty percent of the people who work with computers suffer from visual problems, and forty-nine percent complain about burning eyes. In all probability, young people will spend more and more time in front of a computer as time goes by. And like it or not, we must face the consequences.

Today, the waiting rooms of opticians and ophthalmologists are full of people who are looking for help. For many of them, corrective lenses alone don't provide relief. That is not surprising because we cannot correct vision simply by wearing eyeglasses or contact lenses. Often an existing condition continues to deteriorate, sometimes because of these optical aids.

Many people with visual difficulties, and even those with good eyesight, want to do something to ensure the health of their eyes.

Glasses allow us to live better with our existing visual problems. However, they do nothing to address the underlying cause of the problems.

The Basics of Eye Training

Eyes are an integral part of the human organism. We need to keep that in mind when we treat them.

Experts have designed exercises to address lower back problems. Doctors and trainers use these as part of preventive medicine. The primary focus is on how posture supports the structure of the human body. Among other things, these exercises include lessons in how to lift heavy objects properly, how to sit properly, and how to relax. Instructors teach the participants not to neglect certain muscle groups at the expense of others and not to overly stress muscle groups because doing so can lead to bad posture, chronic tension, and, eventually, to organic damage.

Eye training is based on a similar idea. In this case, we want to establish physical and visual habits that support and stimulate the proper functioning of the eyes.

The Goal of Eye Training

➡ To learn physical and visual habits that support the structure and function of the eye.

➡ To avoid physical and visual habits that lead to eye fatigue, difficulties in accommodation and coordination, overexertion of the eye, restricted or diminished eye movement, diminished field of vision, light sensitivity, night blindness, visual defects, weakness, or injury to the eyes.

➡ To produce dynamic changes in visual function and visual habits and to avoid or overcome limited vision.

➡ To learn how positive external conditions (light, lighting, and nutrition) can promote problem-free vision.

Eye training does not attempt to heal illnesses of the eye. That is a job for an ophthalmologist. Furthermore, eye training is not a therapy that deals with emotional problems, although these often affect the eyes and visual ability. That is a job for an eye specialist, an ophthalmologist who also deals with psychosomatic issues, or a mental health counselor.

Prevention: The Underlying Principle

The goal of eye training is prevention. Eye training stresses countermeasures to use when you've developed bad habits. It also works on proper visual behavior, based on the needs of the eye.

Eye training exercises are easy to learn. You can practice them almost anywhere. They maintain and strengthen your visual abilities, prevent a bad situation from becoming worse, and effectively give your eyes a chance to relax.

Who Should Use These Exercises?

Dynamic, holistic eye training is as useful for people with normal eyesight as it is for those with defective vision, such as those who are nearsighted, farsighted, or cross-eyed. However, people with defective vision should know that the eye training program presented in this book won't reverse their condition. At best, this program might stop a condition from deteriorating, and it might strengthen visual acuity. However, evidence of that does not necessarily show up in lower dioptric numbers.

Eye training is not a substitute for medical examination and treatment! It is simply a valuable tool to reactivate the self-healing powers of the eyes.

See an ophthalmologist for all problems or illnesses involving the eyes. Eye training is not designed to treat illnesses.

Holistic Eye Training

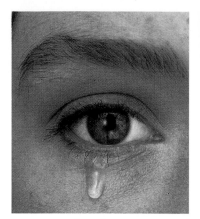

Eyes reflect the emotions and mirror illnesses in the body.

During an eye examination, an ophthalmologist looks primarily at your "optical apparatus" and the internal and external muscles of the eye.

Eye training is based on the holistic concept that the body, mind, and spirit are one.

Seeing with the Whole Body

Seeing is a process of integrating information from the external and physical with the internal and emotional environment. Goethe expressed it this way: "The eyes are the mirror of the outside world and the mirror of the inside of the human being; the totality of the internal and external is made complete through the eye."

The process of seeing involves more than the eyes. You also need the surrounding muscles, the optical nerves, and the visual center in the brain.

To See Not with, but through the Eyes

The energy of the light that falls on the cells of the retina must be multiplied 100,000 times in order for the signal to be strong enough for the neurons in the brain to recognize it as a nerve impulse. The energy itself is available to the whole organism, but it has to be transported to the eyes. In other words, the power of vision comes from the inside. The quantity and quality of external light is very important for good vision. However, regardless of the conditions, the most important factor in the quality of our vision is the sense with which we perceive a visual image.

The Miracle of Vision

"Seeing" is one of the body's most complex activities. Optical information reaches the inside of two dark structures (the eyeballs) through two small openings (the pupils) with the help of light. The lenses, surrounded by muscles that allow for a change in refraction, bundle the information and produce a reversed and upside-down image on the retina of both eyes. Extremely rapid movements of the external eye muscles ensure that both the structures scan the contrast limits of the retina. The optic nerve amplifies and guides the light impulses received. These impulses arrive at a speed of up to 300,000 impulses per second. The optic nerve sends them to the visual centers in the cerebrum, the diencephalon, and the cerebellum.

Nerve Impulses Become Pictures

The recognition of images occurs in both halves of the cerebellum. There, through a scanning process, the information is put together in much the same way that the picture on the screen of a TV set is created with lines. However, the brain works much faster and is able to create a spatial awareness by constantly checking and comparing the information from the left and right eye and by establishing a connection between the two.

Conscious "seeing" is either a recognition or a discovery of something new. Our brains have the choice of comparing the information with images stored in the memory and integrating it into a more or less stable concept of the world, or of using the imagination to see it as a totally new image. We call the latter "viewing."

We know relatively little about what "seeing" is and how it happens. However, scientists are working to solve this mystery.

The Eye:
Cornea (1), Iris (2), Lens (3),
Sclera (4), Choroid (5) Retina
(6), Light yellow dot (7), Optic
nerve (8), Blind spot (9),
Vitreous humor (10), Fovea cen-
tralis (11), Ciliary body (12),
Conjunctiva (13), Posterior
chamber (14), Anterior chamber
(15), Pupil (16)

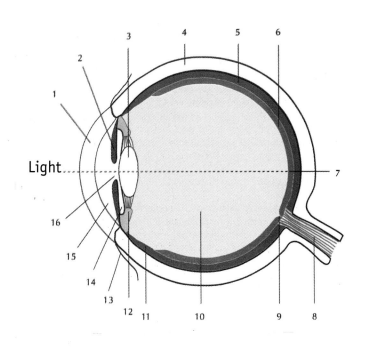

Activities Involving the Whole Organism

From a holistic point of view, the dynamic part of "seeing" involves the whole body, for instance the blood circulation and the organs that detoxify the body. On the other hand, "seeing" also includes an awareness and expression of emotions with and through the eyes and a connection with all the other sensations that enrich and expand visual awareness.

Because we all bring different interests to visual images, we can change visual images. We also can intensify visual images through the joy we experience when looking at beautiful colors and shapes or through empathy. Thus, breathing plays an important role in the holistic concept of the eye because breathing is connected to every emotion and feeling we experience when we "see."

Tension in the Body Affects Vision

Body posture plays an important role in "seeing." Tension can diminish our ability to see.

➡ Clenched jaws indirectly diminish the mobility of the eyes. The nerve that sends impulses from the brain to the eyes, telling them to move, branches out into the jaw, the upper region of the chest, and the neck.

➡ Tense neck muscles diminish blood circulation in the visual centers of the brain, in the eyeballs, and in the eye muscles. Blood flows from the heart through the arteries to the muscles in the neck. From there, it flows to the visual center at the back of the head and to the eyes. Tense muscles in the neck reduce the blood supply to the eyes.

➡ Tension in the back diminishes the field of vision and reduces eye mobility. In order to see properly, the eye, neck, and back muscles must be able to interact.

➡ Tension in the legs, pelvis, and spine can easily diminish muscle balance, the so-called kinesthetic sense. When this happens, a person literally has to hold on to the environment with his eyes because his normal sense of balance is missing.

For example, when your body is relaxed, you can run, walk up a flight of stairs, or walk across an uneven sur-

Since the eyes mirror the overall condition of the body, an eye examination produces information about the state of the entire body.

face, and watch a bird in the sky at the same time. Your legs move automatically on their own.

However, if your body is out of balance because of stress, your eyes try to find support in the environment. You will look in the direction in which you want to move and focus your eyes accordingly. The result is a greatly reduced field of vision, and this puts additional stress on the eyes.

The Mirror of the Soul

We say that the eyes are the mirror of the soul. We experience the truth of this every day when we meet people. Our emotions are obvious in our eyes, and we recognize the same emotions when we look into the eyes of others. Because we are feeling and empathetic beings, what and how we feel directly influences the quality of what we see.

People can have a hard, fixed gaze or a soft, open expression. The hard, fixed gaze speaks of anger and rage. The soft, open look reflects love, joy, and curiosity. The intense emotions generated by fear, unbearable pain, or, at the other end of the spectrum, love, can literally blind us to reality. On the other hand, a lack of emotion conveys a sense of distance and emptiness.

"Seeing" with emotional clarity means that you are able to decide which emotions to express, how much emotion to express, what emotions in the environment you want to react to, and where you need to draw boundaries. In other words, the process of seeing includes the quality of emotional connections, as well as distancing. The quality of emotions and the physical and optical function of seeing create an

Much of the information we receive about a person comes from what our eyes see rather than the words we hear.

inseparable whole. They represent the two sides of the active process of seeing: most emotions are expressed in the body, but physical conditions also affect the soul.

The Mind Recognizes

We "see" or recognize only what we already know. Unless we are interested in what our eyes see, the expression in our eyes remains empty. Experience has shown that eyes become tired much quicker when we have no emotional involvement in our surroundings. Our attitude, our visual ability to remember and imagine, our expectations—all of these play a role in how we perceive an image that appears to our mental eye.

Our mind is constantly perceiving and organizing information even though we are hardly aware of the process.

Consciously Experiencing What We See

According to the French theologian and evolutionist Pierre Teilhard de Chardin, "What is most difficult for humans to see is that which is infinitely far away and infinitely close." The quote emphasizes the point that nothing is more difficult than the ability to "see".

➡ The following exercise will show you "how you see." It is a way of training what your eyes perceive. Do the exercises in a place where you won't be interrupted. Recommended time: ten minutes.

Mirror Exercises

Look in a mirror. What do you see?

1

You see the outside of your eyes:

➡ the front of your eyeballs and the cornea, which covers the round eyeballs like a dome

➡ the white portion of the eyeballs

➡ the pupils, two openings that appear as circular, black holes

➡ the colored iris that gives the eyes their specific color

➡ the eyebrows, eyelids, and the moisture in the eyes

You cannot see the internal structure of the eyes, the surrounding muscles, the optic nerve, and the visual center in your brain. Your sense of vision is like an iceberg in the ocean: you can only see about 1/7 of the total; 6/7 remains hidden under the surface of the ocean. In our case, 6/7 of the visual work is done behind the eyes, inside the head.

2

Now, take a closer look at the visible part and its activities:

➡ The eyes are never still. They move constantly, now gently gliding, now jerking and jumping. They cannot stop, unless forced to remain rigidly focused.

➡ Eyelids blink softly, like a feather or the wings of a butterfly. When they are tired, they feel as heavy as lead, or they jerk nervously. Blinking is completely involuntary unless you deliberately open your eyes wide or squint to narrow your focus.

3

As soon as the amount of light reflected in the mirror changes, the pupils change: they become bigger or smaller automatically. This happens quickly when you are alert and have plenty of light. The reaction is slower when the light is poor or when you are staring at something.

4

Pay attention to the condition of your eyes. Do they look lively or tired, dull or brilliant? Is your expression withdrawn or alert, receptive and focused on the environment or disinterested? Do both eyes look the same or do they appear to be different?

5

Now, become aware of the person that you are looking at, yourself. Are your eyes truly interested in what they are seeing? Do you detect in the expression a focused interest, mental anticipation, or do you see disinterest?

Sadness, joy, pain, rage, love, and isolation are feelings that are like veils. Entire emotional worlds can be hidden behind them. Is the expression in both eyes equal or different?

Mirror Exercises

6

Make eye contact with the mirror image of your own eyes. Look at them. Have a "meeting" with your eyes. As you do, you will see a change in the mirror. The eyes that look at you from the mirror react to what is taking place in your own eyes. The eyes will immediately communicate with the information they receive. Are you looking at your eyes critically or unhappily because they might not tell you what you want to know? If so, you are probably withdrawing even more from what you see.

7

Look at the image in the mirror openly, with curiosity and gentleness. Show understanding if your eyes are under stress. Absorb the feeling of weariness and be ready to do something positive for your eyes, such as a few relaxation exercises. You will notice how your eyes become softer and more open, almost showing anticipation. Look at your eyes with empathy, warmth, and understanding. Have a dialogue with your own eyes. You might realize how unique your eyes really are. Surprise yourself. Learn how much your eyes have to say to you. Don't hesitate to try!

8

Think of eye training as a way to make your "seeing" more animated, using all aspects of your visual abilities. Look in a mirror often, at least once a day. (The best time is in the morning, while taking a bath.) Be open to what your eyes want to reveal to you from the surface and from what the total expression tells you. Become aware that your eyes are a living part of yourself, not just a high-performance organ used to see!

Normally, we use our eyes only to look out at the world. But with a mirror, you can also look into yourself and discover something totally new.

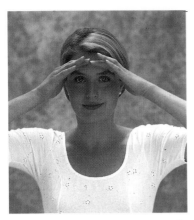

You can improve your eyesight noticeably by doing eye training exercises.

Today's lifestyles make very heavy demands on our eyes, so relaxation exercises are particularly important.

Eye Training in Five Lessons

Lesson 1—Eye Relaxation

Only exercise your eyes when they are relaxed. Otherwise, any exercise might increase tension. Overstressed and exhausted eyes show signs of visual stress: burning eyes, a sense of pressure in or behind the eyes, headaches, twitching eyelids, dry eyes, and occasionally even fuzzy or clouded vision. All of the above may be signs of chronically stressed eyes. If you don't give your eyes a period of relaxation, you can easily damage them further.

Without Force or Pressure

The first lesson starts with relaxation exercises for the eyes (tapping massage) and relaxation exercises for the whole body (stretching and yawning exercises). Eyes that become increasingly moist, perhaps they even shed a few tears, are a wonderful sign that your eyes are relaxed!

➡ Do all the exercises gently and smoothly. Never do them in a jerky or mechanical way. If one exercise is painful or difficult, do not continue it. Stop immediately if you feel any pain or nausea and go to the next exercise.

Exercise 1: A Tapping Massage

You can easily do this relaxation exercise in any position at any time, walking, sitting, or lying down. Recommended time: one to five minutes.

➡ Rub the palms of your hands together. Shake them and rub them as if you were washing them. Then, move one hand over the other, as if you were taking off a pair of gloves.

➡ Imagine that the stress of seeing and of being tired and exhausted surrounds your eyeballs like a crust of clay. Imagine the thickness, color, and density of the clay.

➡ Now, gently tap your fingertips along the edges of the eye sockets, between the eyes (where glasses would rest) and on your temples.

➡ Relax your jaws by exhaling the tension released by the tapping massage. Open your mouth and exhale with a gentle sigh. Then, yawn a few times.

➡ Imagine that the tension, the crust of clay packed around and behind your eyes, is slowly cracking and crumbling .

➡ Continue tapping your forehead, your jaw muscles, and, finally, the back of your head to awaken your visual center.

➡ Continue tapping, moving to the base of the skull, the area between neck and head, and along both sides of the spine. Notice how the tension is slowly melting away.

➡ At the conclusion, gently stroke the areas that you massaged, stroking away from the center of the body.

The tapping massage relaxes the muscles you need for seeing. You'll also notice that your neck and chewing muscles will relax. Recommended time: one to twenty minutes.

Stretch a few times every morning. This will stimulate the circulation and relax the muscles.

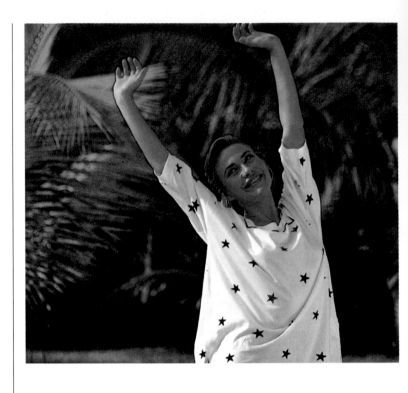

Exercise 2: Stretching

Do these total-body relaxation exercises while sitting. Recommended time: one to five minutes.

TIP
Do the exercise discussed on the right every morning for one to five minutes.

➥ Yawn and stretch your legs, lifting them slightly off the floor.

➥ Spread your fingers and move your left arm as if trying to touch the ceiling with the tips of your fingers. Notice how the left side of your rib cage spreads out like a fan.

➥ Now, reach up as if picking apples. Alternate between looking at the tip of your nose and at your hand, which is reaching towards the ceiling.

➥ Squeeze your eyes shut and playfully wrinkle your mouth. Don't worry, no one is watching! Feel how the muscles around your eyes and neck begin to stretch. Make a clown face or do yoga exercises.
➥ Repeat this whole exercise with your right arm.
➥ Relax.

Exercise 3: Shielding

This is a very simple and effective relaxation exercise for the eyes. Sometimes, people refer to it as optical fasting or palming. Dr. William Bates, the ophthalmologist, suggested this exercise during the 1930s.

The purpose of the exercise is to shield the eyes from all light and to bathe them in darkness. Only eyes that are totally relaxed, closed, and covered with your hands will see a deep blackness.

Memorize the shielding exercises. You'll do them at the end of many of the exercises discussed in this book. Recommended time: one to twenty minutes.

Signs of Visual Stress

People whose eyes are stressed often see fleeting images. These are similar to the images on a television screen after a station has signed off: patterns and colors that move about but often appear gray and diffused. The eyes even mirror mental restlessness. You experience this as swishing images and incomplete darkness when you close your eyes.

Therefore, this exercise is a good way to measure your mental state, as well as your eyesight. When you shield your eyes, the transition from a shimmering, gray state to deep blackness indicates the change from actively seeing to a totally relaxed, restful state.

Only the eyes can experience the sensation of blackness. The feeling produced by this darkness can be of a deep mental rest or of a pleasing sense of mental emptiness, somewhat like diving deep into your inner center, from which essential energy emanates. This can be a deeply relaxing and joyful experience. Do the shielding exercise as often as possible.

Simple Biofeedback

Shielding is a surprisingly simple form of biofeedback. This technique, widely used in research and performance sports, involves expensive instruments which change body signals into acoustic or optical signals.

You don't need any mechanical devices in order to use shielding as a method of biofeedback, and it doesn't cost anything. It provides an excellent way to gauge the degree of tension or relaxation at any time of the day or night.

This exercise deeply relaxes the eyes. After a phase of complete darkness and total relaxation, the vision often becomes surprisingly clear. Colors and contrasts are more lively, and the total field of vision seems clearer, somewhat like the air after a thunderstorm.

We cannot relax on demand. However, we can use some helpful techniques to make it easier to relax.

You can do these exercises:

➡ during a break at work   ➡ while taking a bath
➡ after a meal   ➡ before going to sleep

If you use shielding regularly, particularly after periods of intense work, you will discover a distinct difference in the quality of darkness when you cover your eyes with your hands.

How to Use Shielding

You can do this exercise sitting down or lying down. Assume a comfortable position where nothing will interfere with your breathing. Breathe freely in a relaxed fashion. Recommended time: one to twenty minutes.

➡ Rub the palms of your hands together so that they are warm and charged with energy. Warm, relaxed hands release healing, negatively-charged ions and are very invigorating. Your closed eyes will directly absorb the energy created this way.

➡ Close your eyes. Gently place the palms of your hands over your closed eyes. Rest your fingers on your forehead with the palms of your hands resting on your cheek bones. The palms create a small dome over the closed eyelids. Place the center of your palms over the pupils, without any pressure. Make sure that no light penetrates through your hands.

➡ If you are sitting down, rest your elbows on a table or on your knees. If your are lying down, place a thick pillow under your elbows. Either of these will create a very comfortable position for your hands.

➡ Relax your whole body. Take a few deep sighs—be vocal. Allow your eyes to sink deep behind your closed lids,

The conscious act of inhaling and exhaling plays a very important part in almost all exercises. This deliberate breathing helps you relax and get in touch with your body.

Eye training exercises work as well for people with normal eyesight as they do for those with defective vision. If you wear contact lenses, remove them before starting the exercises.

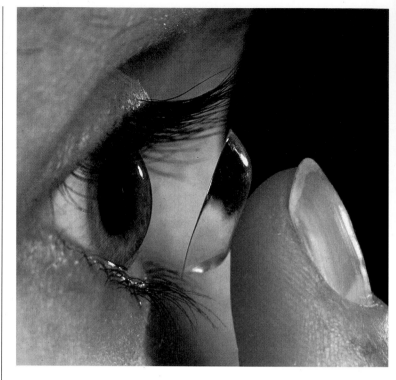

TIP
A simple, but effective way to relax the whole body is to sigh and yawn loudly.

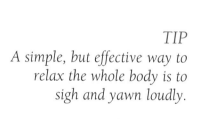

as if resting in a hammock with your head hanging over the edge or into a small, soft lining behind your eye sockets, like sinking into a pillow when you lie on your back.

➥ Be aware of what is happening beneath your closed eyes in the darkness. Do you see anything shimmering, do you see lightening, fog, or patterns? Is the quality of darkness equal or is something moving? Is the darkness more intense in some places?

➥Inhale and exhale deeply. Allow every thought, emotion, and image that appears in the darkness to dissolve every time you exhale.

➥ When inhaling, feel the warmth, the protection, and the touch of your hands through your eyelids and in your eyeballs.

➥ Become deeply absorbed in this process, for at least ten to twenty breaths. When exhaling, observe how the shimmering, pulling sensations; the patterns you see; and the fog enter the darkness and dissolve. When inhaling, allow the energy from your hands to flow into your eyes, filling your eye sockets like a bathtub.

➥ Keep your eyes closed and conclude the exercise by removing your hands from your eyes. Allow your eyes to become accustomed to light again before you open them.

➥ Stretch and bend as if you have just awakened from a nap. Look around. Are your eyes more relaxed and refreshed? Are they interested in what is around you? Has your sense of vision changed in any way?

You can do shielding exercises anywhere. They are very comforting. Do them often!

Important Tips for People Who Wear Glasses or Contact Lenses

➥ Remove your glasses or contact lenses before starting the shielding exercises.

➥ Relax the area around your eyes before starting these exercises. Do short tapping massages with the tips of your fingers (see Exercise 1 on page 19).

➥ Afterwards, look around without your glasses or lenses. Compare your visual impressions with what they were before.

Lesson 2—Refreshing and Strengthening Your Eyesight

The Eyes—Receiving Sunlight

During the course of human evolution, the eyes have developed so that they can use and tolerate sunlight. Their functioning depends on an ideal adaptation to the spectrum of light.

Light is necessary for seeing, but it also goes from the retina directly to the spinal cord and the pineal and pituitary glands in the brain. These glands use it to produce hormones. In addition, cells located deep in the center of the brain receive information from the light and color of the sun. These cells recognize light waves that go beyond the visual spectrum, from infrared to ultraviolet.

Sunlight and color have powerful effects on our subconscious. They greatly influence our well-being and health.

The Function of Daylight

Recent medical research suggests that sunlight influences our biorhythm, alertness and tiredness, our sense of stress and imbalance, and our immune system.

From dawn to dusk, natural sunlight works like natural color therapy:

➡ In the morning, before sunrise, invisible infrared light stimulates our pineal gland and prepares the body for food.

➡ At sunrise, the red and orange spectrum of light serves to rejuvenate and energize us.

➥ At sundown, blue-violet and night-blue portions of the spectrum relax and calm us. The UV-A and UV-B portions of the light spectrum strengthen the immune system and support the healing power of the body. They also stimulate the cells to heal themselves, using light.

Artificial light usually does not have the same qualities as sunlight. In particular, it is missing a well-balanced spectrum. The rhythmic change within its color spectrum is always the same. That lack of change causes light-sensitive cells in the retina and brain to remain in a fixed position. Over time, this can lead to rigidity and to an increased or reduced sensitivity to light. The natural capacity of the eyes to adapt to the total spectrum of sunlight can be lost. The result of such a loss may cause any of the following: increased sensitivity of the lens, difficulty in adapting to sunlight or to light at dusk, night blindness, diminished eyesight, hormonal disturbances, increased tiredness, and seasonal affective disorder (winter depression). The exercise we call "sunbathing" can reestablish the adaptive capacity of all light-sensitive cells in the retina and the brain. This exercise is useful for reinvigorating and strengthening natural eyesight. However, you do need to be careful to avoid being blinded during the exercise.

People in Japan use a sensible method of using sunlight. For some time, they have brought sunlight into living and working spaces with adjustable mirrors.

Exercise 1: Sunbathing

Begin with both of the relaxation exercises from Lesson 1, "Tapping Massage" (see page 19) and "Stretching and Bending" (see page 20). Never look directly into the sun. Don't use sunglasses, prescription eyeglasses, or contact lenses to protect you during the exercise. They only filter out important parts of the spectrum of sunlight.

Sunbathing Without Being Blinded

➡ If possible, choose the gentle morning, afternoon, or evening sun. Avoid the intense sunlight at noon.

➡ Close your eyes! Your eyelids are the best protection against being blinded when you are sunbathing.

IMPORTANT
Before you start sunbathing, please read the instructions at the top of this page.

➡ With your eyes closed, turn your head towards the sun. Relax and feel the pleasant warmth of the sun on your face.

➡ Now, turn your head gently from side to side for about one minute, allowing the sun to completely reach both of your eyes.

➡ Pay attention when you change directions. If your head moves to the left, away from the sun, the light sensors in your eyes move to the right. In other words, they move counter to the movement of your head. If your head turns to the right, the light sensors move to the left.

➡ While moving your head towards and away from the light, observe the distinct change from light to dark beneath your eyelids.

➡ Next, raise and lower your head for about one minute.

➡ With your eyes still closed, move the tip of your nose around the center of the light, first clockwise in a spiral towards the center and then counterclockwise, making the largest possible circle. Continue for about one minute

➡ Next, keep your eyes closed, but expose every part of them to the light for one minute by moving your head any way you like. Each eye has approximately 125 million optic cells, and every one of them would love to catch some of the light.

➡ Finally, cover your eyes with your hands and bathe them in darkness.

Exercise 2: Meadow of Light

After sunbathing, we suggest the following visualization exercise. You can do this during the shielding exercise, and it should take the same amount of time as the sunbathing exercise..

➡ Ask a partner to read or record the text on the following two pages in a quiet voice. (Of course, you may record the text yourself.) Then, invite your optic cells on a journey of imagination.

➡ Assume a comfortable position for shielding. Perhaps you might want to lie down with pillows under your elbows. Relax in this position.

➡ Don't try to will images to come. You may only experience darkness. This is fine. Simply follow the text with your mind or with your other senses. You cannot force the imagination. Images either appear while you are relaxing, or they don't. If images appear spontaneously, and they are not what you expected, accept them anyhow. Feel free to enhance the text we have presented or change it so that it is more to your liking.

➡ Simply let happen what may, without any particular purpose in mind.

When recording the "Imaginary Journey—A Meadow of Light" (see box pages 30 and 31), pass along a copy of this exercise to someone else to use.

Imaginary Journey—A Meadow of Light

You don't have to do anything when you take an imaginary journey, just relax and let it happen.

Lie on your back and relax. Cover your eyes with your hands to keep out all external influences. Cover them completely and gently, as if holding down a feather. Every time you exhale, the tension in your optic cells, dissolved by sunbathing, will fall away and dissipate in the darkness.

With every breath you take, feel the soft touch of protection flowing into your eyes from the palms of your hands.

Imagine a valley, shaped like a bowl, where green grass and beautiful flowers grow. Colorful images blanket the floor of the valley, as well as the retina inside your eyes. Lose yourself, all of your senses and all of your body, in this round meadow of light and color.

Walk through the green, luscious grass. Look at the blue sky which covers the valley like a dome. As you walk, feel the soft grass under your feet and the warmth and energy of the sunlight on your skin. Each blade of grass in the meadow represents a light-sensitive receptor rod in your retina. Each colorful flower in the meadow represents a color-sensitive receptor cone.

Now, walk to the center of the valley, where beautiful flowers grow, just as the cone-shaped cells are organized in the retina. You can find them in the round area that looks like a small crater on the moon. You'll find an enormous amount of flowers here, approximately five to seven million, green, blue, and red in color. They correspond to the three types of

Imaginary Journey—A Meadow of Light

cones which send signals to the brain, allowing us to recognize colors.

Not a single blade of grass grows in this round crater of flowers. Towards the edge of the bowl-shaped valley, the number of flowers diminishes, and towards the edge itself you see only green grass. Walk through this sunlit valley for a while. Enjoy the view of the luscious green, the brilliance of the flowers in the crater, and all the flowers scattered throughout the valley.

Now, imagine watching each colorful flower unfold in the sunlight; watch how each blade of grass stretches towards the rays of the sun.

Feel how each cell in your skin absorbs the comfortable warmth and energy of the sun. Feel how light floods your whole body and flows into every cell.

Feel how your eyes drink in the light reflected from the flowers and grass in the meadow. Observe how light floods the whole valley and the sky above. Feel how walking through the valley recharges your body with gentle vibrant energy, like a battery.

Take one more look at this ocean of flowers and grass before gently and slowly taking your leave. You can return to this meadow after every sunbath. Now, slowly return from your imaginary journey to reality. Take your hands away from your eyes and stretch. Look around and notice how you see the world around you with new eyes.

Each exercise is a remarkable experience which will give you new insight, even if you use it frequently.

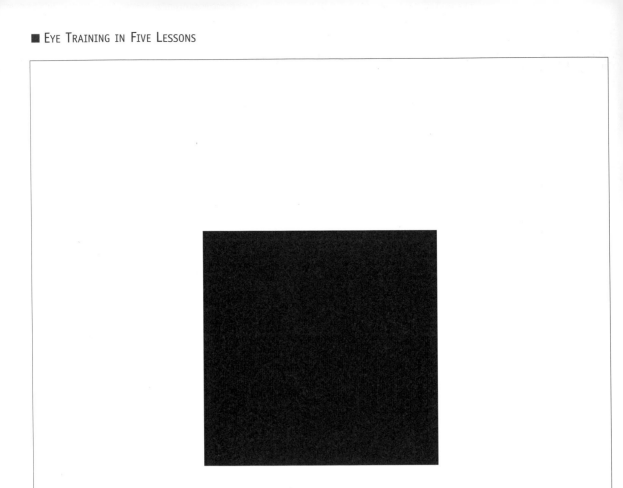

Relax and look at the red surface without glasses. When you inhale, open your eyes wide; when you exhale, return your eyes to normal. Do not stare at the surface. Instead, let your eyes move into the color. Imagine your eyes drinking in the red color.

Exercise 3: Color Bathing

This exercise is an opportunity to learn something about the amazing ability of your visual cells and of your brain: It is your brain, your perception, that produces color and your eyes that radiate these colors! In the process, your eyesight is revitalized and strengthened.

This exercise, called color bathing, is based on an idea of Rudolf Steiner, the founder of anthroposophy. In ancient times, people understood the healing power of color. For instance, in ancient Egypt, they painted certain temple rooms a specific color for therapeutic purposes. Depending on the diagnosis, they sent a sick person to one of these rooms for a healing "temple sleep." They believed that while the person slept, the healing effects of the color were transmitted to the sick person, strengthening the person's own capacity for healing.

Rudolf Steiner, who knew about this ancient wisdom, recommended that people alternate between looking at a red surfce, a gray surface, and finally at a blue surface. Red stimulates circulation in the eyes, and blue aids the body in detoxifying itself. Today, scientific research has confirmed the usefulness of this method. Bathing your eyes in color consists of three interrelated exercises that you should carry out consecutively, one after another.

Set aside ten or fifteen minutes for the whole exercise and try to do them once or twice a day. Use them more frequently during periods of stress.

According to anthroposophic philosophy, colors have symbolic power. Psychologists have confirmed many of Rudolf Steiner's observations with experiments.

Part 1: Bathing in Red

Find a comfortable and relaxed position to sit. Relax your neck and shoulders and breathe quietly and evenly.

After a red color bath, look at a gray surface for about three minutes. You'll probably see greenish or bluish squares. Look at the gray surface until you see only gray with no afterimage.

➡ Place the red square (see page 35) at a comfortable distance from your eyes. Hold it at a 45° angle. Remove your glasses, relax, and look into the red color. The tip of your nose should point to the center of the surface.

➡ When inhaling, open your eyes wide, as if you were trying to expose every optic cell in your eyes to the color. Relax the eyes when exhaling.

➡ Allow the red color to work for about three minutes. Don't stare at the surface. Instead, move your eyes into the color, as if you were diving into a pond filled with a red liquid.

➡ In addition, imagine that your eyes are drinking a red liquid and that the liquid is filling your eyeballs, flowing along the visual pathways to the back of your head, your body, your soul, even to the bottom of your feet.

The color bath should take about two to three minutes. Make sure that you breathe carefully and that you continue to keep your neck and shoulders relaxed. Remain in this comfortable position. Now, slowly move away from the red color and turn to the next exercise.

The different shades that appear in the gray space after you bathe the eyes in red are not accidental. Each color has a specific complementary color. At some point, you may want to experiment with different colors.

Part 2: Bathing in Gray

➡ Next, look at the empty gray surface. What do you see? Are you surprised to see it filled with squares of greenish and bluish turquoise? These are the complementary colors of red.

➡ Look at and into the gray space until you see only gray with no afterimages. Take your time, it might take a while.

Look at the blue surface. Truly dive into the color. Absorb the color as you inhale, just as you did when bathing in red. After two or three minutes, relax your eyes again by looking at the gray surface until no afterimage appears.

Part 3: Bathing in Blue

➡ Next, look at the blue surface. Pretend that you are diving into a pond filled with blueberry juice.

➡ When inhaling, immerse your eyes in the color blue, the same way you did when bathing in red. Don't forget to open your eyes wide when you inhale!

➡ After two or three minutes, relax your eyes by looking at the gray surface again. The orange afterimages won't be quite as surprising now!

➡ Cover your eyes with your hands. After one minute, look at the colors around you. How do they appear now? Are they more vibrant, richer in contrast? If you wear glasses or contact lenses, put them on or in and look around again. Do things look different now? In what way?

IMPORTANT
You can use color bathing as often as you like. The exercise is very balanced, meaning that the tension and relaxation of the optic cells balance each other.

What Are the Effects of Color Bathing?

When you expose your optic cells to gray, the cells assume a state of balance. An equal number of optic cells disperse and receive energy. Experimenters call this process firing or regenerating. This is the neutral state of the retina in which the retina is ready to accept information.

Looking at colors disturbs the balanced state of the optic cells. For instance, when we look at something red, a "red vibration" agitates the color-sensitive cone cells in the retina. When thousands of these cells vibrate, they produce a signal that goes to the brain. The optic cells that have seen the color are exhausted. If you then ask the optic cells to view another color, for instance blue, they have to regenerate very quickly, which means they must return to a state in which they can receive color, the neutral, gray state of the retina.

This process is similar to what happens when a wine taster tastes wine: He always eats a piece of white bread after testing a wine. White bread neutralizes the taste buds and enables the taster to detect the nuance of the next wine.

➡ Try an experiment with water colors. Mix red with its complementary color, green, and you'll have a gray color.

➡ After you expose the brain to red, it quickly sends information back to the optic cells. The information is in green, reestablishing the neutral gray state.

Internal Production of Color

The brain sends the information about color to the retina through the optic path. When you and your eyes are relaxed, the information is projected on an empty surface, just like a slide projector. The internal colors produced by your own sense of vision are among the most beautiful of all colors. While the brain is projecting the internal color to the eye, the flow of energy in the brain is producing alpha waves. This is a state of heightened awareness and mental relaxation. Looking at colors and their complements corresponds to an emotional and mental "receiving" and "releasing." When you are stressed, visually or mentally, you have difficulty seeing colored afterimages. However, after only a few exercises, these beautiful internal images can reappear. Colors and contrasts become clearer and more vibrant.

Color bathing regenerates optic cell activity. These exercises renew the pigment in the optic cells, increasing blood circulation and detoxifying the eyes.

Lesson 3—Eye Movement

In a relaxed state, your eye muscles move up to two hundred times per second. This movement is called a saccade.

Eye movements are normally smooth; however, the more effort it takes for a person to see, the more rigid the movements become. Of course, ease and speed of eye movements are prerequisites for vision. The reason is simple to understand.

➡ Our eyes are only able to focus in a tiny portion of the eye called the fovea centralis. Concentrated in a small crater, this area contains optic cells that focus with razor-sharp precision on black and white and on color contrast. With the help of extremely fast eye movements, the fovea centralis scans the image that comes into the eye through the lens and projects the image on the back of the eye.

➡ After the eye processes the information, the brain creates a clear and complete image. The process is similar to the way a television picture is composed of lines; however, the eye is much more complex because it also includes spatial vision.

Relaxed and Distress Vision

Imagine that your total visual field is one large stage where the background disappears in the distance because of weak lighting. The spot where you can see most clearly is where a spotlight, or in the case of the eyes, the fovea centralis, highlights the area on stage.

If the eyes lose some of their mobility because of stress, the brain automatically switches to an inflexible mode of vision. The brain is trying to compensate for the lack of

TIP
In order for these exercises to be useful for your eyes, they have to have a sufficient amount of vitamins available. You can find the necessary information in publications that deal specifically with the vitamin needs of vision.

mobility by providing more energy so that it can view the largest possible surface of an image and then decipher it.

However, this process is rather stressful, and, over time, it leads to increased tension in the muscles of the eyes and to visual problems.

The muscle movements of the eye, the saccade, are to seeing what chewing is to digestion. In the same way that deliberate and thorough chewing prepares solid food for digestion in the stomach and intestines, soft and relaxed eye movements prepare "visual food" for better recognition by the brain.

Relaxation for Good Blood Circulation

A second reason why relaxed eye muscles are important for our eyes and vision is that the blood supply inside the eyeball is in part provided by the arteries in the eye muscles. If these muscles are distressed because seeing has become difficult, the blood supply diminishes. The result could be metabolic disturbances, such as "floaters," cloudy lenses, or other impairments.

The goal of the following four exercises is to increase the mobility of your eyes muscles. You can practice these exercises standing or sitting. Set aside approximately three minutes for each exercise.

Exercise 1: Eye Yoga

Move your eyes several times from left to right and from right to left. Keep the tip of your nose pointing straight ahead.

➤ Make sure that your eyes are moving, not your head. Are your eyes jumping? Do you see curves or zigzag lines? Allow the movements to become softer and smoother.

Insufficient blood supply and the presence of waste products in the eyes can lead to serious eye illnesses, but you can prevent all of these with exercises.

➥ Breathe and blink your eyes. Relax.

➥ Move your eyes up and down and then down and up several times. Keep your head still as you do this.

➥ Next, move your eyes from left to right and right to left again. Do this several times, keeping your head still.

➥ Move your eyes from the upper corner of the room diagonally to the lower corner. Make sure that the top of your head continues to be parallel to the ceiling and isn't tilting.

➥ Cover your eyes with your hands (see page 23). With your eyes open, "paint" small circles on the palm of your hands. Make a humming sound, like a motor. This stimulates eye movements. Move your eyeballs in both directions.

➥ Keep your eyes covered and closed as you rest for a moment.

Exercise 2: Waggling

➥ Pretend you have a paintbrush attached to the tip of your nose and that you can extend the handle like a telescope. Close your eyes long enough to form a clear picture in your mind of the brush.

➥ Open your eyes and move the brush across the letters of a printed text, pretending that the letters are raised slightly above or indented slightly below the surface of the paper. Pretend you want to dust or polish the letters.

➥ At the end of the line, move the brush back to the beginning of the next line. Imagine that you are painting the white space between the lines with an opaque, white color.

Try to do these exercises regularly. In order to achieve positive effects, you'll have to practice them over time.

➥ Imagine that the polished letters, words, and lines become darker after the brush moves across them but that the spaces between the lines become even whiter.

➥ In this fashion, "read" one paragraph two or three times. Turn the text upside down in order to avoid trying to decipher individual words.

➥ Now, cover your eyes for a while and try to feel the effects of this exercise.

Exercise 3: Swinging

This is an extension of the previous exercise. It deals with your total field of vision.

➥ Look out the window or into the distance. Move the imaginary brush that you've attached to the tip of your nose from left to right. What do you see? Do the bristles touch the horizon? Are you polishing or tickling something?

➥ Move the brush back and forth over the surface of your desk in a very relaxed fashion. Then, slowly bend down, still moving the brush back and forth, until you eventually run the brush across your toes.

➥ Next, trace the outline of your left hand with the tip of the brush. Then trace the lines in your palm. Does it tickle?

➥ Now, change the brush into an imaginary broom. Sweep away everything that you don't want to look at.

➥ Close your eyes and cover them with your hands. Do you still feel the sensation of the movements?

If these exercises are still new and strange, take your time. Practice them slowly and carefully. You can increase the duration and intensity of your exercises over time.

Exercise 4: Accordion

1

Choose something interesting in your field of vision. It should be something that attracts your eyes and that you would like to look at in peace and quiet.

2

First, look straight at the object so that the tip of your nose is pointing directly at it.

3

Frame the object with both hands, the way a photographer would, looking through his fingers.

4

Move your hands farther apart and see what else comes into view. Become aware of colors, shapes, contrasts, movements, etc., in that space. Slowly continue to move your hands farther apart, until they are behind your ears.

5

Move your hands together again, as if trying to touch the object that is the center of your interest.

6

Inhale as you move your hands apart. Exhale as you move them together again. Each time your hands move out, tell yourself, "I give you space." When your hands move together again, say, "I touch you gently."

7

Do these in and out movements as if playing an accordion. Are you experiencing this expanding view emotionally, mentally? Has your visual awareness expanded?

8

Conclude the exercise by slowly reducing the size of the movements.

9

Give your visual senses a short rest by covering your eyes.

Relaxing and resting are as much a part of the exercise program as are attention and concentration. What is important is creating a balance between the two ideas.

Lesson 4—Shifting Between Near and Far Distances (Accommodation)

Swinging and Swaying

Swinging exercises are an easy way to expand your field of vision and to relax your eyes when they are stressed.

Surrender to the swinging, flowing movement while allowing internal images to pass in front of you. Watch the images come and go. Don't try to hold onto them.

Moving yourself and your eyes rhythmically creates a sense of inner harmony. You are letting go of external visual influences. You are finding your center and becoming centered.

Act from Your Center

Your whole body becomes centered when it moves around its vertical axis, the spinal column. When you sway back and forth, the ground supports your weight, so you don't need to "hold on" with your eyes. Your eye muscles are more relaxed, and with the many small vibrating motions, your eyes can dance again, be more alive, be more focused.

In particular, the rotating movement (see Exercise 2 on page 45) gives you a sense of being the center of your environment. You are not looking at the world around you with your eyes but rather looking from a much deeper level through your eyes, and you have a better outlook and can act without getting lost in details.

The midpoint of the arc you create when you swing back and forth is where you find the balance. You can use the following exercises to find your center!

Exercise 1: Swaying

➡ Find a place where you can look into the distance. You might want to look out a window.

➡ Place your feet shoulder-width apart.

➡ Close your eyes. Imagine the movement of a metronome, the instrument that determines the rhythm when you play music, or imagine a windshield wiper moving steadily from left to right and back again.

➡ Now, open your eyes. Your body has become the arm of the windshield wiper or the hand of the metronome, staying very supple and moving from side to side. Your shoulders and arms are relaxed. Your arms hang passively next to your body.

➡ While moving back and forth, softly blink your eyes. Look into the distance without your eyeglasses or contact lenses. Observe how the horizon moves with you as you sway from side to side while everything that is nearby moves in the opposite direction. Become aware of the contrast between what is close and what is far away. Continue this exercise for several minutes.

You can try a variation to this exercise while listening to your favorite music. Try it and see how it feels!

Exercise 2: Rotating

➡ Stand comfortably upright in front of a window. This exercise works best if you remove your shoes.

➡ Form a V with your feet, so that your heels are about the width of your head apart, and your toes are about the width of your shoulders apart.

In the beginning, if you become dizzy, do only the swaying exercise. Don't exaggerate the movements, and stop before you become dizzy. Sit down if you feel dizzy. Put the palms of your hands together and look at your thumbs. You will be surprised how quickly this will cure your dizziness.

➥ Close your eyes. Imagine that a magnet is pulling your head towards the ceiling. This stretches your neck and allows your shoulders to drop. Gently shake your arms to loosen the muscles until your arms hang passively next to your body. Become aware how relaxed you feel.

➥ Take a few deep breaths to become aware of the movement of your abdominal wall and diaphragm. Then, breathe normally.

➥ Imagine that your spine is a string of pearls suspended from the ceiling, running from your head to your pelvis through your feet to the floor. Imagine a hula hoop around your pelvis.

➥ Now, set the hula hoop in motion around this imaginary string of pearls. Make sure you move with your whole body. Open your eyes and let them glide through the environment as if you had a feather attached to the tip of your nose.

➥ Feel how the tip of the feather touches the objects as your eyes move past them. When moving to the right, lift your left heel slightly off the floor. When moving to the left, lift your right heel slightly off the floor.

➥ With each swaying motion, move the imaginary feather up by about the width of one hand. Your eyes will move from left to right and look beyond your shoulders so that you have a 360° view. Don't worry, you won't lose your head.

➥ Don't forget to breathe. When your head touches the back of your neck and the tip of the feather is drawing small circles on the ceiling, start to move the imaginary feather down, the width of one hand with each circular motion, until the tip of the feather touches your toes. Then, continue to swing freely for a few moments more.

➥ As in the case of the swaying exercise or the pendulum exercise, become aware of how objects that are close move in the opposite direction from those in the distance.

➥ Slow down until your body stops moving of its own accord. Don't stop abruptly. Cover your eyes with your hands and enjoy the relaxed and invigorating effect for a little while longer.

Adjustment of Near and Far Vision

Your eyes can adjust to different distances. When they are relaxed, your eyes are able to adjust from very close to very far distances with lightening speed. We call this accommodation.

The muscles that surround the lens of your eye, and to a lesser extent the entire eyeball, perform the accommodation. The muscles are connected to the pliable eye lens through many thin ligaments, in the same way that a round trampoline is attached to the frame with elastic cords. When we look into the distance, the ciliary body muscle expands, flattening the lens. When we look at something close to us, the muscle contracts, just as your lips do when you whistle. This releases the tension in the ligaments, and the lens assumes a dome shape.

The eye lens and ciliary body muscle work closely together. When a lens hardens or the muscles become tense, this cooperation suffers. When you look at something continuously with no real change in distance, for example, at the office where distances seldom vary, your eye muscles become lazy, and this can lead to reduced accommodation.

Your eyes need diversion! If you eyes are always focusing at the same distance, they become tired, This can tighten the muscles and lead to reduced accommodation.

Eye Training Instead of Reading Glasses

When accommodation becomes a problem, the standard answer is bifocals, trifocals, or special eyeglasses for close work. They all make viewing easier at a particular distance. Such visual aids may solve the problem, but they do not address the cause: the loss of a relaxed and broad range of movement between the lens, the ciliary body muscle, the eyeball and the external muscles of the eye.

Age-related farsightedness occurs because the cells of the lens lose their elasticity. The lenses can no longer adjust when looking at something close. When you become impatient, your muscles become even tenser. The tenser they are, the more difficult it is for you to look at things which are close. Then, reading glasses are the only answer. This is not to imply that there is anything wrong with reading glasses. However, you can delay age-related farsightedness with appropriate exercises. You can train yourself to have relaxed, smooth accommodation with the following two exercises.

Exercise 3: Flowing Hand

➡ Sit comfortably on a chair. Move slightly forwards so that your feet support more of your weight. Sit upright. Imagine that a magnet is gently pulling your head towards the ceiling. This will stretch your neck and allow your shoulders to drop. Cover your right eye with your left hand. Keep your eye open under your hand and continue to blink.

➡ Next, move your right hand in a smooth motion in front of your left eye, which is open and blinking. Move it close enough that the image of the hand becomes blurred, and your hand touches your eyebrow or forehead. Next, move your hand away in a wide arc to the right, until it disappears from your view.

Modern bifocals and trifocals make it easy for you to see things that are close and far away. However, this ease presents its own dangers.

➥ While your hand is moving, keep looking at it, focusing on a specific spot, perhaps the ring on your finger or a line in the palm of your hand. Don't try to see everything clearly. Instead of trying to focus, be aware of how the hand becomes blurred as it moves closer to your eyes.

➥ Next, cover your right eye with your left hand. Observe the visual image as the hand moves towards and away from the left eye. At what distance does the hand become blurred? Follow the flowing movement of your hand until it disappears from view behind your left ear.

➥ Play with this movement and alternate between your hands and your eyes.

➥ Conclude by covering both eyes with your hands for a short period of time. Stay with the visual experience.

The "flowing hand" exercise is effective even if your vision is already impaired, and if that is the case, a variety of very specific exercises are available.

Exercises for Defective Vision

AGE-RELATED PROBLEMS

Instead of your hands, use a book for this exercise. Open the book and hold it close enough that your eyebrows touch the page. Observe how the page becomes more and more blurred as it moves closer to your face. Also observe the distance at which the letters become clear again.

Exhale as you move the book towards your face, and inhale as you move it away.

NEARSIGHTEDNESS

Inhale as you move the book towards your face. Exhale as you move the book away. While you are exhaling, imagine that your breath is pushing your hands away.

CROSSED-EYE

Are you or have you been cross-eyed? If so, do the exercises by covering your right eye with your right hand and your left eye with your left hand.

Visual Relay

➥ Position yourself so that you can look out a window. If you prefer, you can do this exercise outside.

➥ Cover your right eye with your right hand.

➥ Choose five or six points to focus on. Each of these should be in a straight line in front of you: The closest will be the tip of your nose, the next will be your index finger, 8–12 inches (20–30 cm) away. For the third point, choose something that is 6–10 feet (2–3 m) away; for the fourth, something 30–50 feet (10–15 m) away. Finally, for the last point, select a point on the horizon.

➥ Let your eyes wander from point to point. Move or jump from one to the next. Remain focused on each point for a little while. Outline each object with an imaginary feather attached to the tip of your nose.

➥ Move your eyes from point to point, forwards and back.

➥ Next, cover your left eye with your left hand. Make the same journey from point to point with your right eye that you did with your left eye. Rest briefly at each point.

➥ Switch between your left and right eye several times, following the procedure outlined above. Your covered eye should continue to blink in darkness.

➥ At the conclusion, "walk" from point to point with both eyes open. Also, look at the tip of your nose with both eyes open. Don't be afraid, you won't become cross-eyed. Actually, cross-eyed means that only one eye follows a movement up close.

➥ Now, cover both eyes and take a few deep breaths. Allow your eyes to relax comfortably beneath the palms of your hands.

Each exercise is an invitation to learn something new. Over time you will find the one you like best and that will become the one that is most effective for you.

Lesson 5—Spatial Perception and Visual Memory

Seeing with Both Eyes

We have two eyes. The two lines of vision cross behind the eyes inside the head. The optic cells inside the eyes guide information to the visual center in the brain.

Modern research discovered that our brain organizes information in two different ways:

➡ The first is the digital method. Here, the brain combines information that is gathered and transmitted separately, such as color, shape, contrast, and movement. The brain combines the information logically, step by step, according to the either/or principle. The brain then compares the image constructed in this fashion with images that are already stored in the visual memory.

➡ The second is the analogous method. Here, the brain combines the same information in an associative, holistic way, according to the "this as well as that" principle. The brain accepts new images spontaneously and interprets them almost playfully, using fantasy, intuition, and emotion. Then, it compares the images to other images it already knows.

Division of Labor in the Brain

In the course of evolution, the human brain became somewhat specialized. The left brain primarily used the logical, digital method; and the right brain primarily used the associative, analogous method. The halves of the brain exchange the results of their activities via the largest "nerve fiber," the corpus callosum. The brain is able to

We construct a complete picture of our world from the visual impression the eyes receive and from the way each half of the brain processes that information. Despite all of their research, scientists are still in awe of this miracle.

integrate these activities so that we are able to receive a complete view of the world. This combined information allows us to view the world from two sides: the logical and rational and the emotional and intuitive.

Optic nerves connect each eye to each half of the brain. That is why someone with only one eye can still switch back and forth between both methods of seeing and comparing. However, both eyes can "see" with both halves at the same time, and two eyes have a greater intensity than one would have. The fact that each eye connects to each half of the brain is what allows us to perceive visual impressions in three dimensions, even though the retina receives them in only two dimensions.

A 3-D computer image gives us a sense of awe about the spatial quality of human vision. The ability to compute a spatial image from information that is centrally and peripherally collected from each eye is astounding. This ability has very little to do with optics; instead, it reveals the enormous work accomplished by our brain.

The difference in the images that the right and left eye deliver produces spatial vision.

Balance Between Activity in the Right and Left Brain

We can easily lose spatial vision when we primarily use our left brain, the part responsible for collecting facts. After all, what is the use of spatial perception when you are trying to organize the images presented while reading a book or looking at a computer? What we don't use becomes weak. For that reason, we shouldn't be surprised that people begin to have problems when they primarily use their visual acuity for left brain vision. However, you can prevent these problems by activating the right half of your brain, training the digital and analogous methods of seeing, and improving the cooperation between your eyes.

Exercises for Spatial Vision

The following three exercises train spatial vision for both eyes.

Exercise 1: Horizontal Eight

➡ Pretend you have a baton attached to the tip of your nose.

➡ Move your head so that the baton "paints" a vertical figure eight, the symbol for infinity, in front of you.

➡ Drop your shoulders and relax. Continue to trace small and large, flat and fat figure eights with this imaginary baton.

➡ Blink your eyes softly and more frequently than usual. Make sure that your neck sways gently with the movement.

➡ "Paint" a horizontal figure eight on windows, doors, objects far away, or simply in the air. Close your eyes and imagine that a paintbrush dipped in your favorite color is swinging from the tip of your nose. Imagine your surroundings covered with colorful horizontal figure eights.

This exercise relaxes your neck muscles, increases blood circulation in the visual centers of the brain, and activates both halves of the brain.

Exercise 2: Finger Frame

➡ For this exercise, you'll use both thumbs. Hold one about 8–12 inches (20–30 cm) away from your nose and the other about 16–36 inches (40–60 cm) away, both in your line of vision.

New techniques make it possible to assist spatial vision with artificially produced 3-D images and even 3-D movies.

The blending of partial images coming from the left eye and the right eye is primarily responsible for creating spatial vision. But other factors also play a role: experience, perspective, shadows, and the fact that with increasing distance, colors become weaker.

➦ If you are nearsighted, focus on the thumb nearest to you; if your problems are age-related or if you are farsighted, focus on the thumb farther out.

➦ Imagine that a bug has landed on the thumb that you are focusing on. In quick succession, alternate between closing one eye and then the other. Is the thumb farther away jumping back and forth, sometimes to the left and sometimes to the right? This indicates that each eye receives its own image, which is different than that of the other eye.

➦ Next, open both eyes and focus on the thumb nearer to you. Can you now see both thumb images at the same time?

➦ Does the thumb "with the bug" appear to be clearer and more three-dimensional than the double image of the thumb farther back?

Congratulations! Your ability to see is equal in both eyes. Each eye receives a picture of the thumbs from a different perspective. The brain is blending the two images into a three-dimensional picture of the thumb that you have focused on. The double image of the thumb that you did not focus on remains two-dimensional because the brain has not blended the images. This exercise makes fusion (or blending) visible, which doesn't occur under normal circumstances.

➦ Now, focus on the other thumb. Does it appear to be framed by two phantom thumbs, as if standing in a doorway? If not, open and close your eyes in quick succession and notice how the thumb jumps back and forth. Alternate your focus a few times between the thumb closer to you and then the one farther away.

➦ At the conclusion, cover your eyes with your hands. Allow them to relax in darkness and give them a short rest.

Exercise 3: Rope Blending

1

Take a rope that is 5 feet (1.5 m) long and tie a series of knots every 4–6 inches (10–15 cm). Attach the end of the rope to a handle on a window, a doorknob, or a shelf that is slightly lower than eye level.

2

Hold the other end to the tip of your nose. Stand or sit so that the rope has no slack.

3

Relax your jaw muscles (try yawning) and your shoulders. Focus on the knot in the middle of the rope, as if a bug had landed there. Allow enough time for both eyes to imagine and see the knot, until a spatial visual impression develops. Are you now seeing two ropes that cross one another at the point of your focus? Does the rope appear to look like an X? If that is case, you are seeing with both eyes, and the blending takes place at the point of focus. If you cannot see an X, blink your eyes again, or in quick succession, use your free hand to cover first one eye and then the other. Can you now see the rope jumping back and forth?

4

Compare both ropes. Each eye sees it differently. What kind of color image is created on the left? What about on the right? How are light and shadow dispersed? What is your visual acuity?

5

With both eyes open, "walk" from one knot to the next. Are you able to take the X along with you? Does an inverted V appear at the end of the rope? Look at the tip of your nose. Do you now see a V?

6

Bend your head forwards. This also bends the legs of the X or V. Play with this forwards and backwards movement. Make yourself larger and smaller and look at the rope. With some training, the rope will look as if a zipper is opening and closing it.

7

Cover your eyes with both hands and rest for a while.

Experiment with different images with your right and left eye!

Exercise for Visual Memory and Imagination

The following two exercises train your short-term visual memory. This memory connects past visual images with new ones that are constantly erased when you blink your eyes. It is also the reason we are seldom aware that our eyelids move.

Don't worry if you remember little of your visual impressions. Remembering too much would unnecessarily stress your visual system, and then you would not blink your eyes enough. You will learn that trying to hold onto everything around you takes effort and is simply not necessary. A well-trained short-term visual memory will give you the confidence to take one look and to remember what you have seen.

Are you a visual person? If so, you can easily store visual images in your memory.

Exercise 4: A Flash over the Shoulder

➡ Stand or sit comfortably with your back to a window.

➡ With both eyes closed, turn your head over your left shoulder. Open your eyes and take a quick look, like a camera taking a picture. As you turn your head back, close your eyes and bring the picture you have just taken with you.

➡ Remember a few of details of what you have seen, such as the background color, a very obvious shape, and a very striking color.

➡ Next, look over your left shoulder with your eyes closed. Take a quick look and immediately close your eyes again. Turn your head back and try to remember a few details.

➡ Do this exercise several times.

➡ Next, repeat the exercise but turn your head over your right shoulder with your eyes closed. Open your eyes and take a quick look again, like a camera taking a picture. Close your eyes. As you turn your head back, take the picture you have just seen with you. Repeating this exercise will provide you with additional details.

➡ With your eyes closed and your head in its original position, try to combine the images you have seen on the right and left into a panoramic picture.

➡ Now turn around and compare the images that you remember with the actual site. How different is it? Is it clearer and richer in detail?

Exercise 5: The Camera

➡ Close your eyes. Then, open your eyelids a fraction of a second, as if taking a picture.

➡ Imagine you have exposed a roll of film in the back of your head. With your eyes closed, imagine the film being developed. Watch how slowly the light-sensitive layer of the film develops into a real picture in a way you have never been conscious of before. What do you see?

➡ Focus your imaginary camera with the lenses set at different distances, from very close to infinity. Mentally examine the developed pictures very carefully. You'll be surprised how quickly the pictures in your memory become clear.

➡ Experiment for a while and then take several pictures in rapid succession. Create a small photo album from your short-term visual memory. Leaf through it, and look at the individual pictures often.

Recalling visual memories is more difficult when you are tired or preoccupied with something else. When that is the case, remember to relax first. Then you can concentrate and do the exercises when you are refreshed!

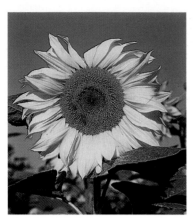

Sunflower seeds contain vitamins and minerals that are important for healthy, good nutrition.

Healthy Tips for the Eyes

Vitamins for Good Vision

The eyes use one-third of the oxygen the heart needs. Although together the eyes and brain represent only two percent of your body weight, during times of stress, they use up more than one-fourth of the energy from your food intake. During times of increased visual demand, for example, from poor lighting or stress, the eyes and brain use far more energy than they would if they were relaxed.

Proper Care for Your Eyes!

The quality of your eyesight depends on the food you eat. This is not just a question of the amount of vitamins. Here, we're also concerned with how your body is able to use them. Your body absorbs vitamins from natural sources easier than from those produced synthetically. However, the vitamins must also be able to get where they are needed, past the blood-brain barrier, located in the back of your head. The vitamins and minerals necessary for healthy eyes must go through the optic channels, the visual center in the brain and the eyes. You can drink as much carrot juice, which contains vitamin A, as you like. If your neck is chronically tense, blood cannot reach your visual centers. The result is that the body stores Vitamin A somewhere else and then eliminates it. Therefore, during times of increased vitamin requirements, we recommend that you use neck massages and eye relaxation exercises as part of your fitness program (see pages 18 to 21).

*VITAMIN SALAD
FOR THE EYE
Ingredients:
1 carrot, 1 apple, 1 lemon, 2
tablespoons sunflower seeds
(outer layer removed), 2
tablespoons vegetable oil
(cold pressed) or cream, 1
tablespoon honey*

*Preparation:
Shred the carrots and apple.
Mix the juice of the lemon,
the sunflower seeds, and the
oil or cream with the honey.
Add to the shredded apple
and carrots.*

Vitamins Your Eyes Need

Vitamin	Importance	Contained In	Nutritional Tips
Vitamin A	To prevent night blindness, to help see in dim light	Liver, parsley, carrots, butter, egg yolk, cod liver oil, and green, leafy vegetables	You can have as much Vitamin A as you want when it comes from natural carotene; one glass of carrot juice a day with a drop of oil is sufficient
Vitamin B1	For light sensitivity	Meat, beans, nuts, wheat germ, potatoes, yeast, and broccoli	About 3½ ounces (100 gm) of steamed broccoli provides two-thirds of daily requirements
Vitamin B2	For light sensitivity	Meat, vegetables, fowl, milk, yeast, soybeans, and eggs	One glass of milk provides two-thirds of daily requirements
Vitamin B12	For light sensitivity	Liver, fowl, fish, meat, eggs, and yeast	Daily requirement is 3mg
Vitamin C	For sufficient blood circulation to the eyes	Citrus and tropical fruit, rose hips, parsley, potatoes, paprika, strawberries, and green, leafy vegetables	Daily requirement is 100 mg; eat fruit and vegetables raw, if possible
Vitamin E	For sufficient blood circulation to the eyes	Oils, seeds and nuts, wheat germ, grain, cold pressed vegetable oils, and green, leafy vegetables	About 3½ ounces (100 gm) of spinach provides one-fourth of daily requirements; sunflower seed oil

Sunflower Seeds

Eating sunflower seeds is an ideal way to give your eyes the vitamins they need. A handful of peeled sunflower seeds a day is, literally, a treatment for the eyes. Be sure that the seeds are free of pesticides and grown organically!

Eye Shower According to Kneipp

The Rev. Sebastian Kneipp, a well known natural practitioner, was absolutely convinced of the natural healing power of water. The eye shower recommended here is based on his method. You can easily include it in your morning and evening ritual.

According to Kneipp, the eye shower increases blood circulation in the parts of the eye exposed to the air. It contributes to the overall well-being of the eyes and strengthens their defense mechanism.

TIP

We recommend eye showers specifically during times of stress and exhaustion, for tired and dry eyes, and when performing intense computer work.

Eye Shower	
IN THE MORNING	IN THE EVENING
With the water running, splash water against your closed eyes fifteen to twenty times	With the water running, splash water against your closed eyes fifteen to twenty times
➡ Start with lukewarm water	➡ Start with cold water
➡ Switch to cold water	➡ Switch to lukewarm water
➡ Conclude by gently tapping your eyes and the surrounding area with a towel	➡ Conclude by gently tapping your eyes and the surrounding area with a towel

Eye Bath

Eye bathing, using a specially designed, oval-shaped cup, cleans the cornea and conjunctiva. It is refreshing and increases the amount of moisture in the eye. It also prevents the eye from burning and becoming red. In addition, it protects the eye from conjunctivitis. Eyecups are available in drugstores and are very inexpensive.

➡ Fill the cup with pure spring water as directed or use water from a filtered faucet. Try to avoid using regular tap water because it is usually too hard.
➡ Place the cup beneath your eye and close both of your eyes.
➡ Bend your head back and press the cup over the socket so that it covers the whole eye.
➡ Blink your eyes so that the water can rinse the front of the eye, including the cornea and the conjunctiva.
➡ Repeat this process several times.
➡ Repeat with the other eye.
➡ Carefully dry the whole area around the eyes with a towel.

We recommend bathing the eyes specifically for people who have a tendency to conjunctivitis or allergies, who live or work in places that are air-conditioned, who work with computers (monitors throw off dust), who live or work in areas of high environmental pollution, and for those who wear contact lenses.

Eye Pillow

Eye pillows are very relaxing. These pillows are usually covered with velvet or silk and filled with the covering from millet seeds that have been grown organically. They absorb static energy, not living, pulsating energy. Thus, they relax the area surrounding the eyes.

➡ First, we recommend that you rest lying down .
➡ Place the eye pillow across your forehead and over your closed eyes. The darkness and pleasant weight of the pillow relaxes your mind and your eyes.

TIP
Eye pillows are available in health food stores. You can also make your own. Create a small covered pillow, about 4 by 8 inches (10 by 20 cm), using velvet or silk. Fill it with millet shells.

Eye Acupressure

Like acupuncture, acupressure is an ancient method used in Chinese medicine. Now, however, it is also widely recognized and approved in the West and all over the world. Acupressure is a type of massage in which you apply pressure with the tips of the fingers. Unlike acupuncture, which uses needles, acupressure requires no instruments. It is an ideal self-treatment technique.

Some of the acupressure points for the eyes are located directly around the eye socket (see photo on page 63). According to Chinese medicine, these points are connected to other organs or organ systems via energy pathways, called meridians. In the case of the eyes, they are the skin, liver, and kidneys. A sure sign that you have found the correct point is a pulsating, sometimes slightly painful sensation. Apply the pressure rhythmically with both thumbs or index fingers at the same time. The tip of the fingers should make small circles over the corresponding acupressure points (numbers 1–3 in the photo). Use light to medium pressure when exhaling and make the circles without pressure when inhaling. Treat each acupressure point for the length of eight breaths.

An acupressure massage helps prevent poor blood circulation of the eyes, cataracts, and glaucoma.

The Effect of Acupressure

Acupressure massage stimulates blood circulation in the front of the eyes, particularly in the sensitive skin around the eyes. It refreshes and energizes the skin in this area. In addition, it relieves and dissolves tension. According to Chinese medicine, since an energy path, or meridian, connects the eyes with other organs, such as

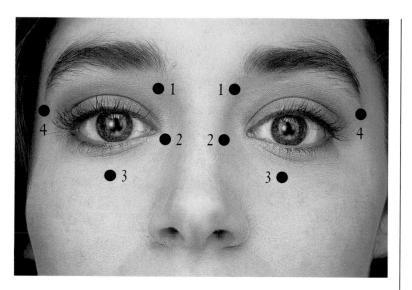

Four important acupressure points are located around each eye: Tian-ying (1), Ying-ming (2), Si-bai (3), and Tai-yang (4).

the skin, kidneys, liver, and stomach, treating the eyes with acupressure can have a harmonizing effect on those areas, too.

➥ With both thumbs, search for the two points identified in the photo as number 1 (Tian-ying points).

➥ During the rhythmical massages, adjust the pressure when exhaling so that you don't create any pain.

➥ If you are not quite sure that you have found the proper point, search a little higher around the edges of the eye socket and the edges of the left and right eyebrow. Acupressure points have an effective radius of about ⅝ inch (1.5 cm), so they cannot be much farther away. After a few treatments, you'll have no trouble finding the proper point.

➥ Massage point number 1 for eight breaths. When exhaling, apply some pressure; when inhaling, release pressure. Rest your other fingers gently on your forehead.

Eye acupressure increases blood circulation and decreases tension in and around the eyes.

Possible Applications of Acupressure

TIAN-YING (POINT 1)

Eye pain from overexertion and tiredness; declining eyesight; pain due to chronic sinus inflammation; colds; and migraines

YING-MING (POINT 2)

Sensitive pressure points from wearing eyeglasses; onset of nose and throat infections; stuffy nose

SI-BAI (POINT 3)

Physical, mental, and emotional exhaustion; toothache; sinus infection

TAI-YANG (POINT 4)

Unspecified headaches, particularly around the forehead; difficulty sleeping because of overwork; eye pain; flickering and pulsating sensations in the eye; high blood pressure

TIP
Acupressure is particularly effective in cases of strained and exhausted eyes and headaches.

Keep your eyes closed and try to feel the effects of the treatment.

➥ Massage both number 2 points (Ying-ming) equally. Use both thumbs or the thumb and index finger of the same hand, pressing rhythmically against the base of the nose for the length of eight breaths.

➥ Feel the effects afterwards.

➥ Massage both number 3 points (Si-bai) in the middle of the lower rim of the eye socket, underneath the opening of the pupil, also for eight breaths. Feel the effects.

➥ Next, place your thumbs at the left and right temples at the number 4 points (Tai-yang). Circle the eyes with the middle joint of the index finger, starting at the base of the nose. Stroke the skin underneath the eyebrows to the outside, back to the base of the nose, down to the tip of the nose, and back again to the base of the nose. Circle the eyes eight times.

At the conclusion, pinch the skin at the base of the nose a few times for one second each, then release.

➥ Place your hands over your eyes for a few moments (see instructions on page 23) and feel the comfortable effects of this massage.

Chinese medicine recommends that you do this massage in the morning and in the evening as a healthy, preventive practice for the eyes. If and when necessary, you may add other massage points to this routine.

Healthy Light

Life could not exist on this planet without sunlight. We need sunlight to see, but our whole body needs it to survive. Nothing equals the natural light of the sun. No substitute is more cost-effective. Eyes are light organs in two respects:

➥ We use a large part of the light we receive for vision through the optic path and the visual nerves.

➥ Another important part of light goes to the hypothalamus and the pituitary glands via the energetic optic path. These glands are responsible for hormone production, the cycle of sleep and alertness, and other biological rhythms. In addition, recent discoveries indicate that they also play an important role in the health of the immune system.

When you need artificial light, try to use forms that imitate sunlight with its spectral components and changing nature. Static artificial light that remains constant might be sufficient for vision, but it is not sufficient for biological functions.

If you consistently spend time in places with artificial light, we recommend that you occasionally change the intensity of the light. If possible, have a dimmer switch that lets you reduce or increase the intensity of the light. A desk lamp or reading lamp should also have a dimmer switch. Use lightbulbs that are as close to the spectrum of sunlight as possible.

Disadvantages of Visual Aids

Many people depend on visual aids. But, sad to say, wearing eyeglasses and contact lenses have their disadvantages.

Lenses Diminish Eye Movement

When your eyesight begins to weaken, eyeglasses provide a remedy. However, eye training might make it possible to improve your vision without eyeglasses.

Optical lenses are cut so that light rays fall at the point of the most exact vision, the fovea centralis in the retina. A person with defective vision sees the total image clearly through eyeglasses or contact lenses, but this means that the eyes no longer have to use the usual small focusing movements to create a sharp image. People with glasses have a tendency to look through the center of their glasses, turning their head rather than moving their eyes. Thus, the area surrounding the fovea centralis usually remains unused. The result is rigid visual behavior. When people remove their glasses or contact lenses, they seem to have a rather stressed expression.

Lenses Prevent Natural Adjustment

According to a study at the University of Münster, natural eyesight for people with normal vision varies during the course of the day by about one-quarter of a diopter. This kind of deviation does not exist for people who wear glasses or contact lenses. If our corrected vision is totally clear, then any positive deviation would actually result in an overcorrection. When we look through glasses that are too strong, we learn how uncomfortable that can be. Since our bodies want to be comfortable, they will suppress any positive adjustment.

In this case, our eyesight loses its dynamics and becomes static and fixed. The advantage is that a person wearing glasses can always see everything in focus. A person with defective vision fails to detect situational deviations. Diminishing eyesight only becomes obvious when we have difficulty focusing. And when that happens, increasing the strength of the eyeglasses becomes necessary. This creates a cycle for those who wear corrective lenses: rigid, stressed, visual behavior causes fixed vision; and this leads to a weakening of the eyesight.

Don't let eyeglasses or contact lenses trap you in a vicious cycle!

Better Eyesight

The goal of eye training is to help people maintain a dynamic balance of visual abilities or to recreate that balance. However, for people with defective vision, this means a more flexible use of corrective lenses depending on a given situation.

The following could be helpful:

➡ Occasionally remove your corrective glasses or contact lenses. When doing so, switch to a softer mode of seeing, enjoying your surroundings, even if they seem blurred. Many artists consciously try to see and create the world around them in new ways by deliberately using their defective vision.

➡ For everyday activities, try to wear a pair of glasses with a weaker prescription (by ten or twenty percent) than you normally use, as long as you don't need to seeing clearly, for instance, to drive. When you supplement wearing these glasses with eye exercises, you might find that your visual ability is changing for the better.

You will soon discover that the weaker eyeglasses will be completely sufficient. Your optician can easily make a pair of these glasses, based on your previous prescription.

In addition, ask your optician for a pair of work glasses, for example, for work at the computer. He will make these glasses to satisfy the specific requirements of your job.

Pinhole Glasses—Pro and Con

These glasses, also called eye exercise glasses, aerobic glasses, or half-tone glasses, are available in many different forms. They have recently become more and more fashionable as "alternative" glasses.

Pinhole glasses are similar to the compound eyes of a fly. They consist of a multitude of small holes in an opaque, nontransparent glass lens. Looking through them gives the wearer a multitude of dot-shaped, sharp picture segments close to one another, without light refraction.

A Simple Optical Trick

The principle underlying pinhole glasses is not new. You can try it for yourself by poking a small hole in a piece of carton and looking through it without any visual aids. In spite of any visual defects you may have, you can see a dot-shaped, sharply focused image. The explanation is that the small hole only allows unbroken light rays to reach the retina through the center of the eye lens. Therefore, the length of the eyeball does not play any role in acuity.

The principle of a camera shutter is the same as pinhole glasses: the smaller the opening, the larger the depth perception.

Pinhole Glasses

ADVANTAGES

➡ They stimulate quick eye movement because the eyes move from hole to hole. In this way, the wearer collects individual pieces of visual information that the brain combines into a total image.

➡ Eye muscles move easier and blood circulation in the eyes improves.

They prevent or correct visual rigidity.

➡ Saccadic movements for minute adjustments of the eyes increase.

➡ They stimulate accommodation of the lenses and ciliary body muscles.

➡ Spatial perception at the periphery does not change when compared to refraction lens, which means space is not distorted.

➡ The complete range of light reaches the inner eye through the small holes, even though the amount of light is greatly diminished.

➡ Pinhole glasses are a very sensible alternative to sunglasses.

DISADVANTAGES

➡ The eyes do not receive a complete and clearly focused image.

For that reason, you cannot use pinhole glasses when driving a car.

➡ You will need some time to become accustomed to pinhole glasses. We recommend that, in the beginning, you wear these glasses for only a few minutes every day. Increase the duration slowly over time.

➡ At dusk and in case of poor light conditions, the light reaching the eyes is too low.

➡ For these reasons, pinhole glasses are not a true alternative to prescription eyeglasses. However, because they exercise your eyes, they most certainly can help you to relax them, which is also very important. In addition, they can also increase visual mobility.

Fashion, gag, or serious alternative to corrective lenses? Whatever the case, a pair of pinhole glasses is surely a novel solution for visual problems.

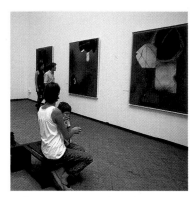

The exercises in this chapter are designed to increase your visual perception.

The exercises are meaningful preventive measures for the health of your eyes, but they may also provide very interesting new experiences.

Eye Training with Posters

By now you are already familiar with the eye training program that lets you coordinate and strengthen your vision. The last chapter dealt with healthy tips for the eyes, using simple and effective preventive measures.

This chapter shows you how to use posters to train your visual behavior and abilities.

Keep These in Mind for All Exercises

➡ Sit comfortably and keep your shoulders and neck relaxed.

➡ Imagine that a magnet is gently pulling your head up from the center towards the ceiling.

➡ Hold the page at a comfortable distance. You don't need to see everything in sharp focus. If possible, hold the picture at a point between where it would be focused and where it becomes blurred.

➡ If you have defective vision, do the exercises without wearing your glasses or contact lenses.

➡ Hold the book so that the page is at a 45° angle and the tip of your nose points to the center of the page.

➡ Relax, breathe, and blink your eyes frequently during the exercise.

➡ Don't forget to shield your eyes for a few moments after every exercise in order to intensify the effects.

Exercising Your Perception of Contrast

Poster: "Dotted Screen"

The exercise using the dotted screen (see page 73) strengthens your ability to perceive contrasts. It trains your eyes to focus on one point, exercising focused vision. The three exercises that follow can also improve your visual acuity.

Exercise 1

➡ Invite your eyes to take an impromptu walk across the picture. Are all the black dots equally intense, or do some appear to be darker than the others?

➡ Let your eyes jump to where the black color seems to be the most intense. That might be a dot you are looking at, a dot in a different spot, or several dots in several different places.

➡ Let your eyes jump to the point that seems to be the darkest as quickly or as slowly as you want.

Black and blacker. These are completely subjective impressions.

Exercise 2

Look at the total picture and choose one particular dot you want to focus on.

➡ Wait until a brilliant white edge appears around that dot like a neon light or like something illuminated from behind.

➡ Does the black color of the dot now look darker than before and darker than the black of the dots next to it?

➡ Now look at a different black dot. Pay attention to your breathing: breathe through the dot. Open your eyes wide when you inhale and try to inhale through the dot. Relax your eyes when exhaling, as if to use your eyes to breathe out through the black dot. Can you still recognize the white edge around the dot? Is that edge even brighter than before?

➡ Let the flow and the rhythm of each breath connect you to the dot you are looking at. Always stay with each dot long enough for the brilliant white edge to become intense and for the dot to appear to be framed by a neon light.

Recommended time: one to two minutes.

The dot screen represents an evenly constructed pattern, but your eye also creates visual impressions.

Exercise 3

➡ Pretend you have a paintbrush attached to the tip of your nose and that you are painting effortlessly and without pressure. The brush should easily follow each movement of your nose.

➡ Pretend that the black dots on the screen are slightly raised above the white surface or slightly indented below it.

➡ Pretend that you are carefully and smoothly applying rich white paint around the black dot that you are looking at.

➡ Repeatedly dip your imaginary brush into the brilliant white paint.

➡ Now, imagine you are using black ink. Dab the dot you are looking at with black ink and outline the edge of the dot with the ink.

Recommended time: one to two minutes.

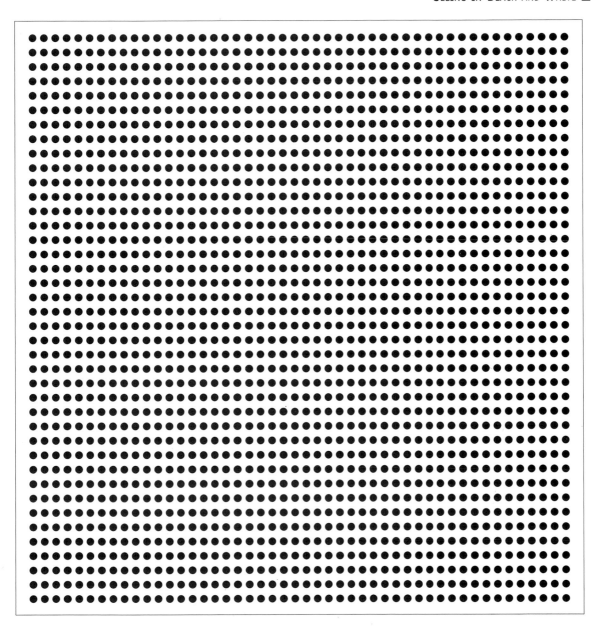

1. Allow your eyes to wander spontaneously across the dots. Always look at the dot that seems to be the darkest. 2. Imagine that you have a paintbrush attached to the tip of your nose. Paint a white ring around the dot that you are looking at. Recommended time: one to two minutes.

Exercising Eye Movement

Poster: "Maze"

The "maze" exercise is a way of training your eyes to follow a prescribed figure or object with smooth movements. This exercise is a wonderful opportunity to train your eye movement, and good eye movement is indispensable for relaxed reading.

As an aside, the maze on the next page is an outline of a very unusual landscaping plan from Pimpern, in the British county of Dorset. Rose hedges frame the path through the maze. This type of landscape was very fashionable in the seventeenth century and early eighteenth century. The drawing on the right comes from an engraving dated 1758. It was prepared from a drawing by John Bastard. Here, you can walk on a path lined with rose bushes, at least with your eyes.

➡ Follow the path of the maze with your eyes.

➡ Imagine you are following the tracks of a quickly moving ant.

➡ Make sure that you are relaxed, that you breathe calmly and deeply, and that you blink often.

➡ Your neck muscles must participate in the movement. Pretend that a line runs from the tip of your nose to the imaginary ant moving in front of you. With small movements of the tip of your nose, move the ant like a puppet through the winding path.

Recommended time: one to five minutes.

The maze is a classic problem-solving exercise. Eye movement has a great deal to do with solving this type of task.

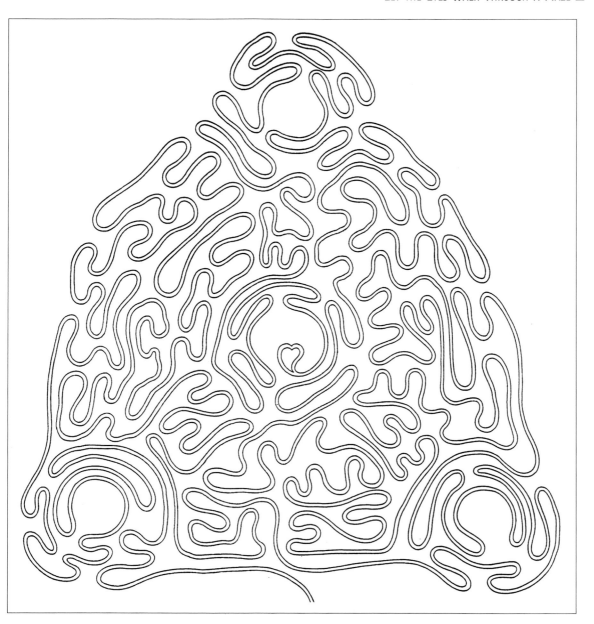

Follow the path through the maze with your eyes. Imagine that a rope connects the tip of your nose to an ant that is walking ahead of you. With small movements of your nose, push the ant through the path. With your eyelids, imitate the steps the ant is taking.

Training The External Eye Muscles

Poster: "Visual Jumps"

This exercise strengthens the outer eye muscles. These muscles determine the ability of the eyes to move quickly from one point to another, to interpret an object quickly, and to move on to the next image. The two exercises strengthen visual orientation and improve the speed of recognition.

The eyeball is surrounded by six muscles which allow the eyes to focus in different directions.

Exercise 1

➡ Focus on point A. Jump to the next point and then from point to point until you reach point B.

➡ Remain at each individual point for one breath and allow your eyes to relax there. Use your peripheral vision to anticipate the next point before your eyes jump.

➡ Only then go on to the next point.

Exercise 2

➡ Start at point B and slowly guide your eyes from point to point until you reach point A. Use your neck muscles, adding a dot of paint to each point with the imaginary brush attached to your nose.

➡ Once you reach point A, quickly jump from point to point again, until you reach point B.

➡ Now, starting at point B, jump two points forwards and one point backwards until you reach point A.

Recommended time: one to three minutes.

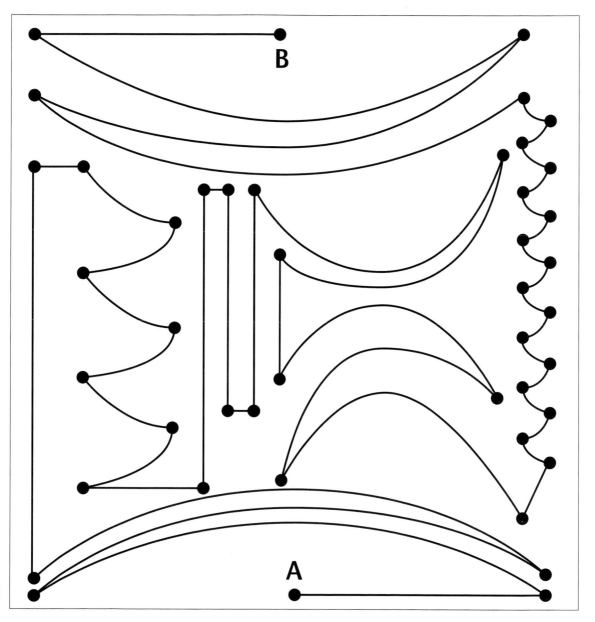

Focus on point A. Let your eyes jump to the next point, remaining there for the length of one breath. Then, allow your eyes to go to the next point. Rest there. Continue until you reach point B.

Exercising to Relax the Eyes and to Improve Visual Perception

Poster: "Flower of Light"

This exercise is a light meditative relaxation for the eyes that helps with the perception of whole objects. The exercise to improve perception involves all of the senses.

➥ Take a look at the drawing. Absorb the total image; let it speak to you.

➥ Experience its centering effect as if your eyes were trying to nestle into the shape.

➥ Let your eyes be drawn to the center.

➥ Expand your field of vision with complete awareness and imagination. Start at the center of the picture and move to the outside. Take in one whole colorful ring at a time. Notice the way the ring moves around the center.

➥ Continue to work on increasing your field of vision. Move from the center to the outside in stages, until you see the shape and its surroundings as a whole.

➥ Now, move back to the center, letting your eyes jump from ring to ring. Relax, breathe deeply, and blink your eyes frequently.

➥ Again, move from the center out with relaxed eyes until you become aware of the "flower of light" in its totality.

➥ Relax and take in the image as a whole with softly focused eyes. Become aware that all of your senses are involved. Do you perceive a pulsating movement in the image? Let yourself be surprised and enjoy the effect.

Recommended time: five to twenty minutes.

In everyday life, our eyes must recognize visual signs and symbols quickly. Viewing something with relaxed eyes that focus on the total image provides the necessary balance.

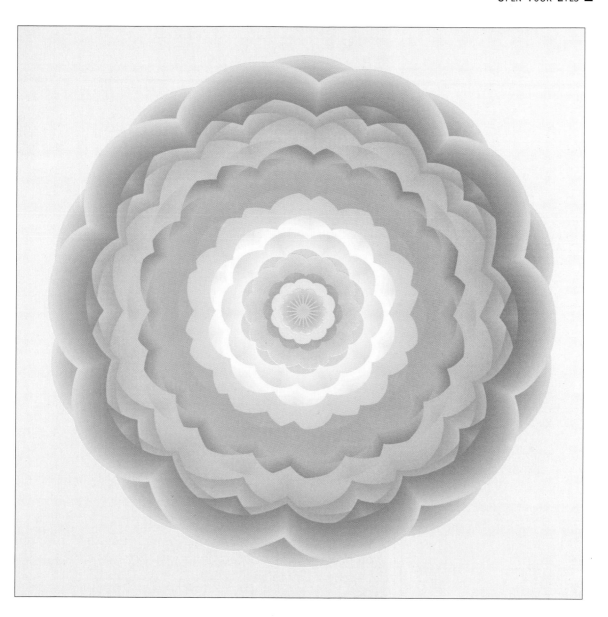

Allow the image to enfold you. Let your eyes dive into its center. Open your eyes wide, let your eyes jump from ring to ring, and return again to the center. Breathe deeply, blink your eyes often, and become aware of all the other sensual impressions.

Exercising Close Vision— Accommodation

Poster: "Letter Size"

Exercise 1

➡ Cover your right eye with one hand. Don't apply pressure. During the exercise, continue blinking the eye that is covered. Hold the page with the text vertically in front of you with the other hand.

➡ Focus with your left eye on a word in the first paragraph. Now, with or without glasses or contact lenses, move the text close to the eye until the word becomes blurred. Move the text away from your eye and then move it so close to your eye that the word disappears completely.

➡ Continue with this in-and-out movement, which is like playing a trombone.

➡ Next, cover the left eye. Continue the near and far positions of the text until the word you are focusing on totally disappears.

➡ Go to the next paragraph and repeat the exercise with each eye.

➡ Move on to the third and fourth paragraphs and repeat the exercise for each eye.

Recommended time: one to two minutes.

Exercise 2

➡ Imagine that you have a paintbrush attached to the tip of your nose. Move the imaginary brush over the letters of the first line of the first paragraph. Imagine that the black letters are raised off the page and that you are using the brush to dust them.

A trombone player alters the tone his trombone produces by changing the slide with jerky in-and-out movements, lengthening and shortening the slide. You'll use similar jerky movements to change distances here.

If the eye would not be like the sun, the sun would never see it. If God's power did not reside within us, how could that which is divine delight us? Johann Wolfgang von Goethe

I am not asking for magic and vision, Lord, but only to have the strength to live life everyday. Teach me the art of small steps. Make me resourceful and give me imagination so that in the daily helter-skelter of life I may take note of the discoveries and experiences that I meet.

May I have a sure sense of the proper allotment of time. Give me the gift of instinctive knowledge so that I may know what is first and what is second. Give me the strength to be disciplined and to show moderation so that I may not drift through life but arrange each day sensibly. Help me to recognize rays of hope and the highlights in my life so that I may, now and then, find time for pure enjoyment. Make me aware that dreams change nothing, neither the past nor the future. Help me to do the next thing I have to do as best as I can and to recognize this hour as the most important in my life. Protect me from the naive belief that everything in life has to go smoothly. I ask for the gift of sobering knowledge that I may accept that difficulties, losses, mishaps, and relapses are the free and natural gifts of life which help us to grow and mature.

Remind me that the heart is often in conflict with logic. At the right moment, send somebody who has the courage to lovingly tell me the truth. I ask that I may always give You and everybody else the opportunity to speak. Truth is not what I proclaim it to be but what is told to me. I know that many problems are solved by doing nothing. Give me what I need to wait. You know how much we need friendship—give me what I need so that I may be worthy of this most beautiful, most difficult, most risky, and most gentle gift. Give me the necessary imagination to deliver a small package filled with kindness at the right moment, with or without words. Make me into a person who is like a ship with great depth so that I may also reach those who are "below." Protect me from the fear that I may miss something in life. Give me not what I want, but what I need. Teach me the art of small steps! Prayer of Antoine de Saint-Exupéry

Focus on a word anywhere in the text with one eye and cover the other eye. Then, move the text close to your eye until the word starts to become blurred. Move the text away and then close your eye again. Continue this movement, which is similar to playing a trombone.

➥ At the end of each line, move your imaginary brush between the lines to the beginning of the second line. Then move from left to right.

➥ While the brush is moving back between the lines, become aware of the letters in the lines above and below, as if they were telephone poles flashing by the window of a moving car.

➥ Work yourself through the next three paragraphs the same way. Do not try to recognize everything. On the contrary, it is helpful when the letters are not clear, even when they become blurry.

Consciously blending individual images received by the left and right eye often creates surprising effects. Try it and see what your eyes might produce.

Exercises to See with Both Eyes

Poster: "Color Fusion"

➥ Hold one finger midway between the tip of your nose and the picture. Look at the finger with both eyes, not at the picture. Do you see four images in the background, two blue and two red?

➥ If not, in quick succession close one eye and then the other while still looking at your finger. Do the two dots in the background jump to the left and then to the right?

➥ As soon as you see the images jumping, look at your finger again with both eyes, and, with a bit of patience, you will be able to see the four images in the background.

➥ Now, move your finger towards the tip of your nose until the double image of both dots in the background shifts and you can see three images.

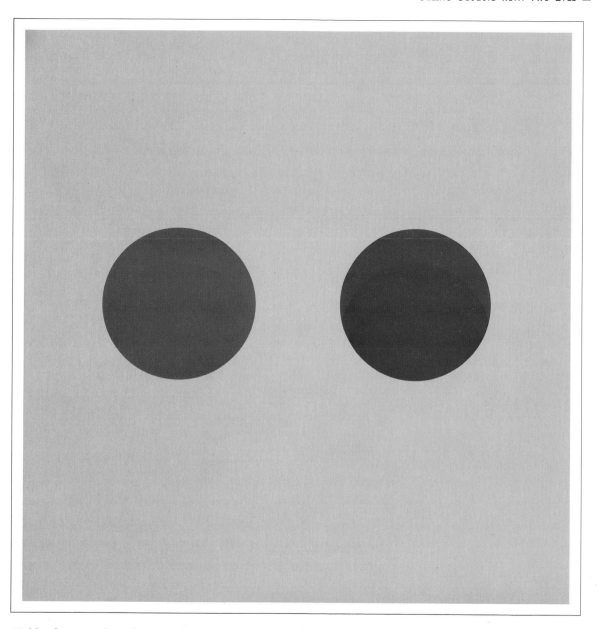

Hold a finger midway between the tip of your nose and the picture. Look at the finger. Can you see four partially overlapping color images in the background? If not, try quickly closing one eye first and then the other. Do the images jump back and forth in the background?

Observe and enjoy the kaleidoscope of colors during this blending process. Does it remind you of a shimmering opal?

➡ If both eyes see with equal intensity, violet, a secondary color, will appear. You can change the kaleidoscope of colors by focusing on one color, for instance red, and then on another color.

➡ The presence of a harmonious, dynamic kaleidoscope of colors in the area of blending, where the secondary color is most brilliant and the dot seems to be suspended in space, is a sign that the fusion process in your brain is active and receiving energy.

➡ You will be mentally centered and visually more present and open afterwards. Alpha wave activity in your brain increases, and this is a sign of a relaxed and receptive state.

Recommended time: one to five minutes.

If you are unfamiliar with the magic of 3-D-pictures, this exercise may take a little while. Be patient, eventually you will see it, too!

Exercising Stereoscopic Vision

Poster: "3-D Picture"

While they challenge us with their magical charm to find hidden spatial structures behind the surface, 3-D pictures also have a healing effect. They are relaxing when we are involved for too long in concentrated, one-sided vision. They also stimulate 3-D perception and imagination.

➡ With both hands, move the picture close to your face and then away again.

➡ When moving the picture away, look with unfocused eyes through the picture as if looking through colored glass.

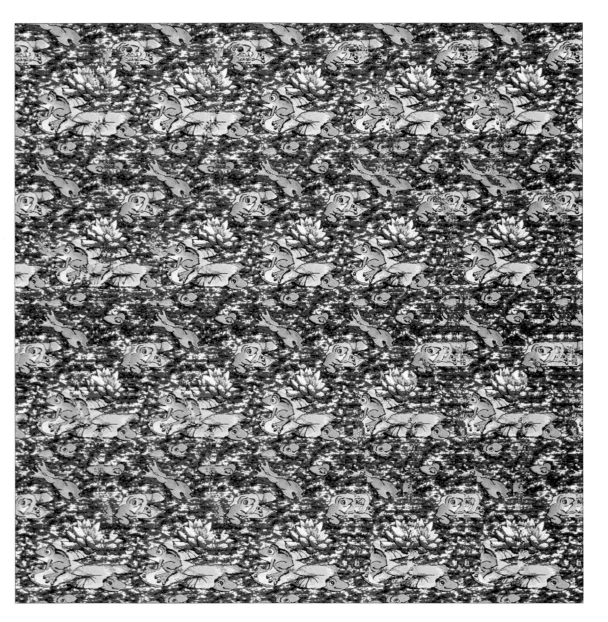

Move the 3-D picture close to your face and then slowly away again. When moving it away, look through the picture with unfocused eyes. It is okay if the images begin to blur. After a while, a 3-D image will develop that your eyes can walk through.

➥ It is perfectly okay if the images become blurred.

➥ If, as the picture is moving away from your face, a 3-D picture does not appear spontaneously, repeat the process several times, like the "trombone playing" in Exercise 1 on page xx.

➥ Relax as soon as a 3-D image appears. Let your eyes walk through this image. Imagine walking around the 3-dimensional structure and in the space surrounding it. Become aware of how spatial impressions slowly begin to deepen and widen.

Recommended time for beginners: one to five minutes. For those more experienced: ten to twenty minutes.

The "landscape" exercise will give you some ideas about your short-term visual memory while you exercise it.

Exercising Visual Memory and Vivid Imagination

Poster: "Landscape"

This exercise trains your eyes to provide a quick, accurate, and detailed comprehension of pictorial information. The two exercises will increase your short-term visual memory.

Exercise 1

➥ Take your time, relax, and look at the photo.

➥ Close your eyes and try to imagine the picture with your inner eye. Let your imagination color the photo like a picture in a child's coloring book.

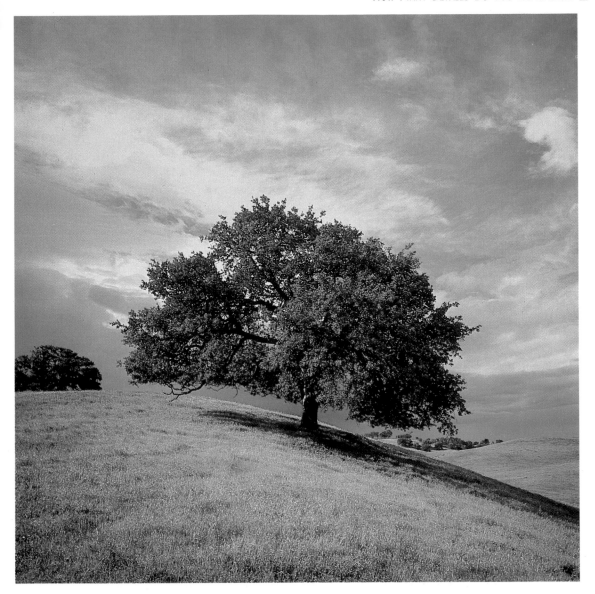

Take your time, relax, and look at the photo. Close your eyes and try to see the picture with your inner eye. From memory, color the photo in your mind. Then, open your eyes again. Which of the surfaces and colors did you remember?

➡ Open your eyes and take a look at the landscape photo again. Which of the details did you remember? Which colors?

Exercise 2

➡ Hold the photo in front of you and close your eyes.

➡ Quickly open your eyes for a fraction of a second, as if taking a photo.

➡ Imagine that your brain is developing the picture you just took of the photo. With your eyes closed, imagine it developing. Watch how the contours slowly become clearer and sharper. Take your time. Then, look at the finished picture in your mind.

Recommended time: one to two minutes.

Exercise 3

➡ Take your time and look at the photo.

➡ Close your eyes.

➡ In your mind, place yourself into the landscape.

➡ Listen to the sounds around you. Smell the fragrances in the air and take a walk through the setting.

➡ Imagine what the environment looks like past the edges of the photo. Immerse yourself in that part of the landscape.

➡ Try to find a beautiful place that invites you to linger for a while. Enjoy your stay in this place.

➡ Now, turn your attention to the real world again. Open your eyes and stretch your limbs as if you just woke up from a nap. Take another look at the photo to see how your imagination has expanded it.

A picture provides a huge, complex mass of information. Each viewer chooses different information and, in that way, composes his own "picture," according to his short-term visual memory.

Short Exercises for Lively Vision

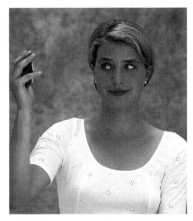

The following twenty simple exercises are healthy exercises for your eyes. Practice them daily.

Eight Steps to Success

Many exercise programs fail because they take up too much time. Our short exercise program tries to avoid this pitfall. Although you'll only need a little time, two or three minutes for the whole program, it is extremely effective, particularly when you do it several times during the day.

The program consists of twenty exercises that you do consecutively. The individual steps are easy to learn, and most of them you already know from the five lessons (pages 18 to 57).

Establish a regular schedule for your daily exercise program. Your eyes will be grateful for the consistency.

Daily Comfort for Your Eyes

Do all of the exercises gently, smoothly, and playfully. Never use jerky or mechanical movements. Should one exercise be painful or difficult for you to do, don't force yourself. Conclude the exercise as soon as you feel pain and go on to the next exercise. Breathe deeply as you exercise. If you hold your breath or use shallow breaths, which often happens when you are exerting force or effort, the area you are trying to stretch won't receive enough oxygen and will become stressed. Exhaling cleanses the body, expelling toxins. Make sure when you

Short Exercise Program in Eight Steps

1

Relax and concentrate as you do the following exercises.

2

First, read through the text. You will see that the exercises are easy.

3

Go through all of the exercises once.

4

Make a commitment to do four of the twenty exercises from memory at least four times during the day. The first day do exercises one through four; the second day, exercises five through eight; the third day, exercises nine through twelve; the fourth day, thirteen through sixteen; and the fifth day, exercises seventeen through twenty.

5

Once a day, do all twenty exercises consecutively. Use the book to help. You will find that the exercises flow easily.

6

On the sixth day, begin increasing the exercises daily. The sixth day do exercises one through eight consecutively; on the seventh day do exercises one through twelve; the eighth day, one through sixteen; and the ninth day do all twenty exercises.

A Tip: Copy the relevant pages from the book; this makes it easier when you need to look up an exercise.

7

From the tenth day on, make sure that the transition from one exercise to the next is smooth.

8

You'll enjoy this program more if you find one, two, or even more people to exercise with you. One person could be the leader.

IMPORTANT!

You can do these exercises sitting down or standing up. You can do them at work or at home. People who spend long hours working at computer terminals need short rest periods, which would be the prefect time to exercise.

Remove your eyeglasses and your contact lenses when you exercise.

exhale that you do so totally. Keep your mouth slightly open, then inhaling becomes automatic.

Twenty Quick Exercises

Exercise 1

Look to the left and inhale. Hold the tension in the muscles of your eyes and count to three. Exhale. Look straight ahead again. Take a deep breath and relax.

Exercise 2

Look to your right and inhale. Hold the tension in your eye muscles and count to three. Exhale. Look straight ahead again. Take a deep breath and relax.

Exercise 3

Look at the ceiling and inhale. Hold the tension in your eye muscles and count to three. Exhale. Look straight ahead again. Take a deep breath and relax.

Exercise 4

Look down and inhale. Hold the tension in the eye muscles and count to three. Exhale. Look straight ahead again. Take a deep breath and relax.

Exercise 5

Turn your head to the left, look over your left shoulder, and inhale. Hold the tension in the eye muscles and count to three. Exhale. Turn your head and look straight ahead again. Take a deep breath and relax.

Exercise 6

Turn your head to the right, look over your right shoulder, and inhale. Hold the tension in the eye muscles and

If possible, open the window during the exercises so that you get plenty of fresh air.

count to three. Exhale. Turn your head and look straight ahead. Take a deep breath and relax.

Exercise 7

Fold your fingers behind your head. Push your head down, but continue to look straight ahead and inhale. Hold the tension in the eye muscles and count to three. Exhale. Raise your head again, look straight ahead, and relax completely.

Exercise 8

Rest your head on your fist with your chin pushing into the fist. Look straight ahead and inhale. Hold the tension in the eye muscles and count to three. Exhale. Take a deep breath and relax the neck and the whole body.

Exercise 9

Move your eyes to the left for as long as it takes for three breaths. Quickly close your eyes, relax, and take a deep breath.

Exercise 10

For the length of three breaths, move your eyes to the right. Close your eyes, relax, and take a deep breath.

Exercise 11

For the length of three breaths, use your eyes to trace a huge vertical figure eight on the opposite wall. Close your eyes for a moment, take a deep breath, and relax.

Exercise 12

Raise your arms and push both hands to the sides three times. With your eyes unfocused, look between your hands. Close your eyes, take a deep breath, and relax.

After each exercise, you must relax. You won't get the desired effect it you omit this very important step.

Exercise 13

Cover your right eye with your right hand and place your left thumb in front of your face, about 16 inches (40 cm) from the tip of your nose. Look towards the horizon, at your thumb, at the tip of your nose, at your thumb again, and finally at the horizon (see "Visual Relay" exercise on page 50). Close your eyes, take a deep, long breath, and relax.

Exercise 14

Cover your left eye with your left hand. Hold your right thumb 16 inches (40 cm) from the tip of your nose. Look towards the horizon, at your thumb, at the tip of your nose, back to your thumb, and then towards the horizon again. Close your eyes, take a deep breath, and relax.

Exercise 15

Hold one thumb 8 inches (20 cm) from your face, the other 16 inches (40 cm) away. Both should be on the same level. For three breaths, look at the thumb closer to you. Become aware of two images of the thumb in the background (see "Finger Frame" exercise on page 53). Close your eyes, take a deep breath, and relax.

Exercise 16

Place your thumbs in the same position as in exercise 15, but focus on the thumb farther away from you for three breaths. Become aware of the image of a frame in front of you. Close your eyes, take a deep breath, and relax.

Exercise 17

Yawn loudly and heartily three times.

Exercise 18

For the length of three breaths, move your lids very fast, like the wings of a humming bird.

Our sense of vision is naturally inquisitive. Support the intensity and liveliness of your eyes!

Exercise 19

➥ Let your eyes wander (see "Waggling" exercise on page 41).

➥ For the length of three breaths, enjoy the contrast of light and shadow.

➥ For the length of three breaths, enjoy the variety of color around you.

➥ For the length of three breaths, observe the different shapes around you.

➥ For the length of three breaths, become aware of the different movements in your field of vision.

➥ For the length of three breaths, expand your field of vision.

Exercise 20

Gently stroke your eyes and the area around them for the length of three deep, relaxed breaths. Cover your eyes with both hands and bathe them in darkness (see "Shielding" exercise on page 21).

This whole short exercise program only requires a few minutes. You should take time out every day for the health of your eyes.

About the Author

Wolfgang Hätscher-Rosenbauer has a Master's Degree in Education, and is a Gestalt and color therapist. He is the director of the Institute for Visual Training in Bad Vilbel, Germany, and conducts courses in Germany and abroad. The eye-training program was developed and is presented by him as a course for preventive medicine.

Disclaimer

The content of this book has been carefully examined. However, neither the author nor the publisher assumes responsibility for any possible negative results or damage resulting from the advice contained in this book

Photo Credits

Dominik Parzinger, Munich: 18, 89; IFA. Taufkirchen: Title page (Ostarhild), 58 (E. Pott); Südwest Archiv, Munich: 12; The Image Bank, Munich: 20 (Curto); Tony Stone, Munich: 1 (John Lund), 6 (Terry Vine), 10, 63, (Paul Dance), 24 (SBHA), 70 (A. Merola), 87 (Carr Clifton).